A Holistic Approach to Organic Synthesis

Synthesis is one of the distinguishing features of chemistry as a science. It is the synthetic chemist who uses their intimate understanding of molecular structure and properties to produce materials of great value to society. Thus, it is important for students of chemistry to study synthesis and acquire a working knowledge that enables them to address the following question: given a specific molecular target, how does one formulate a plan for its synthesis? This synthesis primer provides students who have taken introductory organic chemistry with a set of tools that can be used to plan a synthesis. It may be used in conjunction with a synthetic methods course, or it can stand alone.

Features

- Provides students who have taken introductory organic chemistry with a set of tools that can be used to plan a synthesis.
- Serves to help organic chemists at all levels to better understand published syntheses.
- Focuses on natural products, their complexity, and diverse structures that challenge and inspire the chemists preparing them.
- Succinct, readable treatment of important concepts and applications geared toward advanced undergraduates and graduate students.
- Each synthesis covered begins with a brief discussion of the target molecule and challenges they present and is followed by retrosynthetic considerations.

A Holistic Approach to Organic Synthesis

Philip Garner

Professor of Chemistry, Emeritus
Washington State University, USA

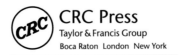

CRC Press
Taylor & Francis Group
Boca Raton London New York

CRC Press is an imprint of the
Taylor & Francis Group, an **informa** business

Front cover images: bioravenShutterstock, DeCe/Shutterstock, notbad/Shutterstock, The Author.

First edition published 2024
by CRC Press
2385 NW Executive Center Dr, Suite 320, Boca Raton, FL, 33431

and by CRC Press
4 Park Square, Milton Park, Abingdon, Oxon, OX14 4RN

© 2024 Philip Garner

CRC Press is an imprint of Taylor & Francis Group, LLC

ISBN: 978-1-032-43923-5 (hbk)
ISBN: 978-1-032-43843-6 (pbk)
ISBN: 978-1-003-36943-1 (ebk)

DOI: 10.1201/ 9781003369431

Typeset in Times
by Deanta Global Publishing Services, Chennai, India

Contents

Acknowledgements

I would like to thank my family and friends for their support and encouragement throughout the course of this project. I am especially grateful to my loving wife, Andi, for keeping me focused and making everyday life seem normal as I navigated through the stages associated with the preparation of this book. I am indebted to the following individuals who read through my drafts and made substantive comments and suggestions: Ryan Joseph (Washington State University), Nicholas Sizemore (University of Scranton), Jin Cha (Wayne State University), Casey Cosner (MilliporeSigma), and my good friend Mike Smith (University of Connecticut).

Preface

Synthesis is one of the distinguishing features of chemistry as a science. It is the synthetic chemist who uses his/her intimate understanding of molecular structure and properties to produce materials of great value to society. No aspect of our everyday life has been left untouched by chemical synthesis. Thus, it is important for serious students of chemistry to study synthesis and acquire a working knowledge that enables them to address the following question: given a specific molecular target, how does one formulate a plan for its synthesis? This primer is intended to provide students with a set of tools that can be used to plan a synthesis.[1] In recent years, we have seen how chemistry departments have increased the diversity of their curricula. This is generally good! However, students wishing to specialize in organic synthesis are often short-changed as a result, such as, for example, when graduate courses are no longer offered on a regular basis so that new courses in other important areas can be taught. In the context of organic synthesis, the "traditional" curriculum for an organic chemistry student included a physical organic course, a synthetic methods course, a total synthesis course, and a sprinkling of more specialized mini courses or seminars. This is simply not possible in many departments today. This book is my attempt to address this problem by giving students a good foundation in synthesis that can be taken to the next level with or without taking the full complement of "traditional" courses.

Computer programs that combine expert systems and artificial intelligence (AI) recently succeeded in designing synthetic routes to some moderately complex natural products.[2,3] Are the resulting syntheses truly innovative and an improvement over prior art? This gets to the crux of the AI issue: how does one think creatively about organic synthesis? In Reference 3, the human-proposed use of an apparently unrelated rearrangement was the key innovation that resulted in a concise (three-step) synthesis of the alkaloid stemoamide. Seeing the connection between a known rearrangement and the target structure is what a creative human synthetic chemist does. In any event, these AI achievements beg the question: will the study of synthesis by humans still be relevant five years from now? This is a valid question. At the present time (2023), the short answer, in my humble opinion, is "yes," as computers cannot yet be truly creative in the sense that "creativity" implies inventing something that has never been done before. Coming up with something novel is difficult with well-known targets that have been synthesized by multiple groups. One approach to creativity involves asking what portion of the target molecule's structure you would like to make without focusing on viability. The results are often flawed, but there is usually a germ (gem?) of an idea in the mix that often leads to the invention of a new method that becomes part of the synthetic plan. One can then move on to addressing potential problems and plan optimization.

Even if future technical advances see the emerging AI technology applied to complex molecules routinely, preparation of the target is only one of the goals of the synthetic endeavor. The study of synthesis necessarily inspires creative thinking that, in combination with logical thinking, leads to invention. In this way, synthesis stokes the fires of discovery. Finally, the study of synthesis serves as an excellent training ground for future generations of chemists, providing them with an unparalleled skillset for employment in either academia or the industrial arena. A brief note about my choice of content: in keeping with its intended purpose, this volume is not exhaustive in its coverage of published syntheses. Specific syntheses have been chosen for their didactic potential—or because they are favorites of mine! As expected, any opinions expressed are my own.

About the Author

Philip Garner received his PhD from the University of Pittsburgh under the guidance of Paul Dowd. This was followed by postdoctoral training in Paul Grieco's laboratory at Indiana University. In 1983, he took up his first faculty position at the Illinois Institute of Technology in Chicago. He moved to Case Western Reserve University in Cleveland, Ohio in 1985, where he established a research program that focused on methodology for the synthesis of bioactive molecules. In 2007, he moved across the country to join the Department of Chemistry at Washington State University. Over the course of his career, Dr. Garner has trained more than 50 undergraduate researchers, graduate students, and postdoctoral fellows. He has published more than 100 papers. His scientific accomplishments include the development of a widely used serinal derivative that has come to bear his name. He currently holds the rank of Professor Emeritus.

Introduction

The focus of this book will be on the synthesis of natural products and their analogues that, because of their diverse structures, challenge and inspire the chemist who wishes to prepare them. A primary goal of early synthetic chemists was to prove the structure of a natural product by synthesizing it in the lab using robust functional group keyed reactions and establishing identity of the synthetic substance with the natural product. This rationale for synthesizing natural products has largely been replaced by modern spectroscopic methods and X-ray crystallography (though structural assignments continue to be corrected by synthesis). Today, natural product synthesis also serves as a theater to "field test" new synthetic methods by demonstrating their practical application, to provide a basis for medicinal chemistry and drug development, and to foster creative thinking as noted in the preface.

The synthetic chemist may be considered a molecular architect of sorts, as he or she designs a viable and detailed plan to build a complex molecule using available synthetic technology. One may draw an analogy between target-oriented synthesis and the game of chess. In both chess and synthesis, a particular problem can be analyzed in terms of (1) a goal to be achieved (synthesis of target = checkmate), (2) a fluid strategy to be followed (evolving synthetic plan = evolving game plan), and (3) tactics used to implement the strategy (specific reactions = individual chess moves). However, the analogy breaks down if one considers the standard "moves" that one must choose from. In chess, the moves available to each piece are constant and have not changed over time. Having made this comparison, it is interesting to note that one of the pioneers of modern synthetic planning, Robert Robinson, coauthored a book on chess.[4]

New chemical reactions, on the other hand, continue to be developed, and they evolve over time as new technologies become available. The sophistication and quality associated with your final synthetic plan will likely depend on the number of reactions that you have in your "toolbox." Thus, it is important to build up this personal resource as you proceed in your studies. I believe that the best way to do this is to try to study total synthesis papers, looking up concepts and reactions that you are not familiar with, and writing out working mechanisms for each reaction used. Each chapter will focus on the planning behind the synthesis of selected natural products or structurally related analogues. Reactions that you may not be familiar with will be accompanied by a succent description and working mechanism in "soft boxes" along with lead references. Each chapter will include a short tutorial and a set of practice problems that reinforces concepts that were introduced. To set a baseline for this book, it is assumed that you have learned the concepts and reactions listed below in your introductory organic chemistry course. You should review any concepts or reactions that you are not fully familiar with before you start Chapter 1.

CONCEPTS

1. Lewis structures
2. Resonance
3. Tautomerization
4. Arrow pushing
5. Molecular orbitals
6. Orbital hybridization
7. Frontier molecular orbitals
8. Reaction coordinate versus energy diagrams

C–C BOND FORMING REACTIONS

1. Alkylation of acetylide anions
2. Grignard reactions
3. Aromatic substitution
4. Enolate chemistry
5. Aldol addition and condensation
6. Claisen condensation
7. The Wittig reaction
8. The Diels–Alder reaction

FUNCTIONAL GROUP INTERCHANGES

1. Acid-base reactions
2. Reduction of alkenes and alkynes
3. Hydroboration/organoborane oxidation
4. Dihydroxylation of alkenes
5. Epoxidation of alkenes
6. Halogenation of alkenes and alkanes
7. Reduction of carbonyls
8. Dissolving metal reductions
9. Alcohol oxidations
10. Ester and amide formation
11. Imine and enamine formation

As discussed in the preface, there is an element of creativity involved in synthesis that is often easier to appreciate than to quantify. As in chess, a good way to learn the game (i.e., how to plan a successful synthesis) involves analyzing the work of masters. This will be our approach as we study selected syntheses performed by master chemists. Each synthesis covered will begin with a brief discussion of the target molecule and the challenges it presents, followed by retrosynthetic considerations, and, finally, a discussion of the key aspects of the synthesis that was performed, noting problems that were encountered along the way and their solution. Each chapter will include a list of reactions that were used but that you may not be familiar with.

Some of them will be described in more detail in the chapter. You should look up these reactions on your own,[5] familiarize yourself with them, add them to your reaction toolbox, and use them when you work on the practice problems. Many reactions simply go by the name of their inventor or discoverer (for example, the Sharpless asymmetric epoxidation), so you should become familiar with those named reactions that are commonly used either by searching the internet or consulting a dedicated reference book.[6] But before we start our journey, we will review some basic synthetic concepts and describe in detail what we have termed as the holistic approach to synthesis.

REFERENCES

1. A book that focuses on how to make disconnections and that provides many examples and problems is: Warren, S., & Wyatt, P. (2008). *Organic synthesis: The disconnection approach*. John Wiley & Sons.
2. Mikulak-Klucznik, B., Gołębiowska, P., Bayly, A. A., Popik, O., Klucznik, T., Szymkuć, S., ... Grzybowski, B. A. (2020). Computational planning of the synthesis of complex natural products. *Nature, 588*(7836), 83–88.
3. Lin, Y., Zhang, R., Wang, D., & Cernak, T. (2023). Computer-aided key step generation in alkaloid total synthesis. *Science, 379*(6631), 453–457.
4. Robinson, S. R., & Edwards, R. (1973). *The art and science of chess: A step-by-step approach*. Harper & Row.
5. A good reference book that you can use to look up reactions which you are not familiar with is: Smith, M. (2016). *Organic synthesis*. Academic Press.
6. Kurti, L., & Czakó, B. (2005). *Strategic applications of named reactions in organic synthesis*. Elsevier.

List of Abbreviations

Ac	acetyl
AD	asymmetric dihydroxylation
AIBN	azobisisobutyronitrile
All	allyl
Aux*	chiral auxiliary
BBN	9-borabicyclo[3.3.1]nonyl
BHT	butylated hydroxytoluene
Bn	benzyl
Boc	*tert*-butoxycarbonyl
Bu	*normal*-butyl
Bz	benzoyl
Cbz	benzyloxycarbonyl
Cp	cyclopentadienyl
dba	dibenzylideneacetone
DBU	1,8-diazabicyclo[5.4.0]undec-7-ene
DCM	dichloromethane
DDQ	2,3-dichloro-5,6-dicyano-1,4-benzoquinone
DEAD	diethylazidodicarboxylate
DIBAL	diisobutylaluminum hydride
(DHQD)$_2$-PHAL	hydroquinidine 1,4-phthalazinediyl diether
DHP	dihydropyran
DIP	diisopinocampheyl
DME	dimethoxyethane
DMF	dimethylformamide
DMP	Dess-Martin periodinane
DMSO	dimethylsulfoxide
DMPU	*N, N'* - dimethylpropyleneurea
dppf	1,1'-bis(diphenylphosphino)ferrocene
HMPA	hexamethylphosphoramide
Ipc	isopinocampheyl
KHMDS	potassium bis(trimethylsilyl)amide
LAH	lithium aluminum hydride
LDA	lithium diisopropylamide
LDBB	lithium di-*tert*-butyl-biphenylide
MCPBA	*meta*-chloroperbenzoic acid
Mes	mesityl
MOM	methoxymethyl
Ms	methanesulfonyl
NHK	Nozaki-Hirama-Kishi
NIS	*N*-iodosuccinimide
NMO	*N*-methylmorpholine-*N*-oxide

PDC	pyridinium dichromate
Ph	phenyl
pin	pinacol
PMB	*para*-methoxybenzyl
PPTS	pyridinium *para*-toluenesulfonate
pyr	pyridine
Red-Al	sodium bis(2-methoxyethoxy)aluminum hydride
sp	sparteine
TBAF	tetrabutylammonium fluoride
TBDPS	*tert*-butyldiphenylsilyl
TBS	*tert*-butyldimethylsilyl
TEMPO	(2,2,6,6-tetramethylpiperidin-1-yl)oxyl
TES	triethylsilyl
TFA	trifluoroacetic acid
Tf	trifluoromethylsulfonyl
THF	tetrahydrofuran
TPAP	tetrapropylammonium perruthenate
Ts	toluenesulfonyl

1 A Simple Holistic Approach to Planning a Synthesis

BACKGROUND READING

- **Historical view of modern organic synthesis** (Seeman, J. I. (2018). On the relationship between classical structure determination and retrosynthetic analysis/total synthesis. *Israel Journal of Chemistry, 58*(1–2), 28–44.)
- **Retrosynthetic thinking and analysis** (Corey, E. J. (1988). Robert Robinson lecture. Retrosynthetic thinking—essentials and examples. *Chemical Society Reviews, 17*, 111–133.; Corey, E. J. (1991). The logic of chemical synthesis: multistep synthesis of complex carbogenic molecules (Nobel lecture). *Angewandte Chemie International Edition in English, 30*(5), 455–465.)

PRELUDE

The commercial production of organic compounds touches every aspect of our lives. Here is an example that involves the development of antiviral drugs to treat influenza (Figure 1.1). One of the stages in the virus's life cycle involves the cleavage of a terminal sialic acid residue located on the surface of the infected cell by the viral enzyme neuraminidase. Oseltamivir (Tamiflu) is a commercially available synthetic drug that binds to the viral enzyme's active site, thus antagonizing the enzyme's function. The resulting change in host cell surface morphology inhibits release of the newly formed virus particles from the host cell. The drug is manufactured (i.e., synthesized on a very large scale) from the natural product shikimic acid, which can be harvested from the spice known as star anise or produced by fermentation using genetically modified bacteria. Such "small molecule" drug-based therapies complement immunization (for example, the annual "flu shot"), which may not be feasible for patients with compromised immune systems.

Unfortunately, oseltamivir is not effective against COVID-19, which is caused by the SARS-CoV-2 virus and is responsible for the current pandemic that plagues the world. This state of affairs has spawned efforts by multiple pharmaceutical companies to develop an effective antiviral drug that targets COVID-19. Pfizer's drug Paxlovid (which contains PF-07321332 also known as Nirmatrelvir, which is the structure on the left in Figure 1.2), an antagonist of the main SARS-CoV-2 protease that is essential for COVID-19 replication, was approved by the US Federal Drug Administration (FDA) for the treatment of mild to moderate COVID-19 infections.

DOI: 10.1201/9781003369431-1

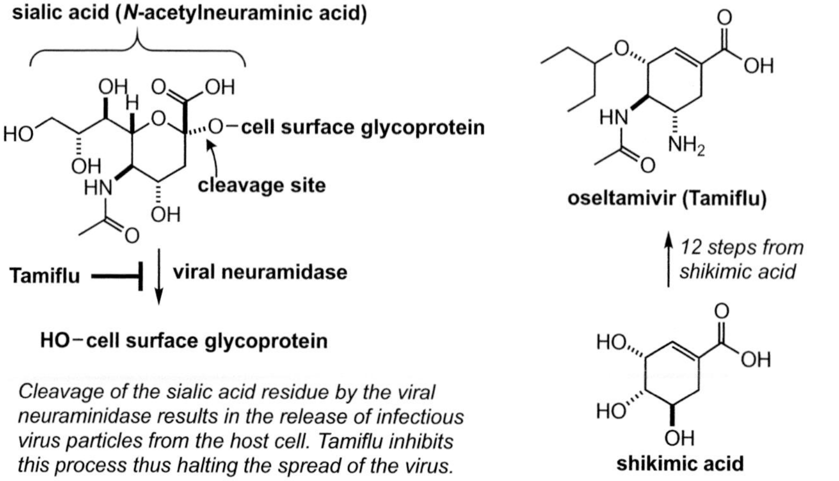

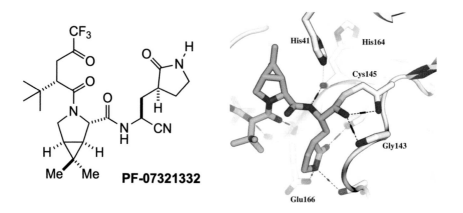

sialic acid (*N*-acetylneuraminic acid)

oseltamivir (Tamiflu)

Tamiflu ⊣ **viral neuramidase**

12 steps from
shikimic acid

HO−cell surface glycoprotein

*Cleavage of the sialic acid residue by the viral
neuraminidase results in the release of infectious
virus particles from the host cell. Tamiflu inhibits
this process thus halting the spread of the virus.*

shikimic acid

FIGURE 1.1.   The molecular target of the flu virus neuraminidase and its mode of action
(left). The structure of the synthetic neuraminidase inhibitor oseltamivir (also known as
Tamiflu) along with the starting material used for its commercial synthesis (right).

PF-07321332

His41   His164

Cys145

Gly143

Glu166

FIGURE 1.2.   The molecular structure of Nirmatrelvir (left) and its covalent structure
bound to the SARS-CoV-2M^{pro} protein (right). X-ray crystallography was used to determine
the 3-dimensional structure of the addend formed when Nirmatrelvir binds to the enzyme's
active site. Only part of the protein structure is shown, labelling the amino acid residues that
interact with the drug. (The 3-D image is taken from Reference 1.)

Nirmatrelvir was chosen from a group of lead compounds as the clinical candidate based on ease of synthetic scale-up, enhanced solubility that facilitated formulation, and reduced propensity for epimerization. The covalent binding of Nirmatrelvir
to the protease's active site cysteine residue via addition of a nucleophilic thiol to the
electrophilic nitrile is shown on the right (minus hydrogen atoms).[1]

How Would You Go About Designing a Chemical Synthesis of Tamiflu or Nirmatrelvir?

The development and commercialization of drugs such as Tamiflu and Paxlovid involves the combined efforts of teams of scientists from different fields, with organic synthesis playing a critical role in the process. From a didactic point of view, it is instructive to consider how one might synthesize complex molecules such as Tamiflu or Nirmatrelvir. A prospective solution, in which one builds a complex molecule from simpler precursors in a stepwise manner, is not so obvious! What molecular building block would you start with? What reactions would you use to add molecular complexity? Later in this chapter, we will revisit the Nirmatrelvir synthesis problem in order to teach students how to develop a synthetic plan using this molecule as an example. We consider our step-by-step approach to be ***holistic*** in the sense that it involves comprehension of a molecule's structure, physical properties, reactivity, and reaction mechanisms.

Let's Begin by Defining Strategy and Tactics

Strategy – The art of devising plans or stratagems toward a specific goal.

In the context of organic synthesis, strategy equates to a plan for the synthesis of a target molecule. The plan may be detailed but must be fluid, meaning that it is modifiable if problems are encountered during its execution. It is prudent to have a contingency plan ready in the event that a problem turns out to be insurmountable. The strategy must also consider constraints such as the time frame or the required quantity of the final product.

Tactic – The art or skill of employing available means to accomplish an end.

The tactics used to support a synthetic strategy correspond to the chemical reactions that are used in organic synthesis. Not surprisingly, the more chemical reactions one has in their reaction toolbox, the more sophisticated the synthetic plan can be. Reactions that do not require expensive equipment, reagents, and solvents are preferred as are those that do not produce a significant waste stream. This last point is related to the concept known as green chemistry, which encourages chemists to design chemicals and chemical processes in a way that avoids the creation of toxic substances and waste (https://en.wikipedia.org/wiki/Green_chemistry).

Now Let's Review Some Basic Reaction Concepts

- **Substrate** – The starting molecule (or molecules) upon which a particular reaction is to be performed.

- **Reagent** – A summary of the experimental conditions one applies to the substrate to accomplish the desired conversion.

- **Product** – The molecule (or molecules) resulting from the action of the reagents upon the substrate.

- **Chemoselectivity** – The selective action of a reagent on one of multiple functional groups.

There are two functional groups in the substrate: a carboxylic acid and alkene. The Fischer esterification reagent, which is shown, selectively acts on the carboxylic acid and not the alkene.

- **Protecting groups** – Temporarily mask the normal reactivity of a functional group.

In this example, there are two functional groups in the substrate, a carboxylic ester and a ketone. Selective reduction of the ester is desired. However, the ketone is more reactive than the ester. A strong nucleophile, such as lithium aluminum hydride, will react with both the ketone and the ester producing an undesired diol. Therefore, the ketone must be "protected" as a ketal resulting in the desired chemoselectivity. As a result, two additional steps (protection and deprotection) are added to the reaction sequence.

- **Regioselectivity** – The selective action of a reagent at one of multiple sites on a molecule.

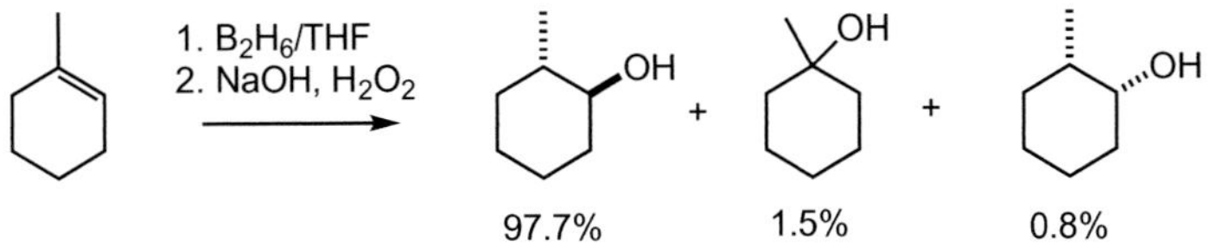

97.7%   1.5%   0.8%

There are two nonequivalent carbon atoms in the trisubstituted alkene of 1-methylcyclohexene. Hydroboration occurs selectively, primarily in an anti-Markovnikov fashion, installing the hydroxyl group preferentially at the less substituted carbon after oxidative rearrangement of the intermediate organoborane species.[2]

- **Stereoselectivity** – The selective formation of one stereoisomer in which more than one is possible.

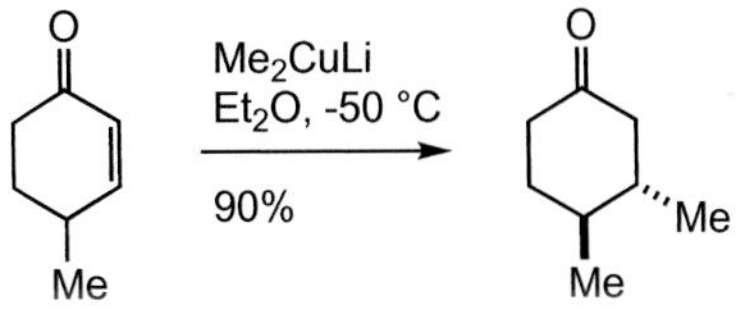

In this diastereoselective reaction, the organocuprate reagent adds to the less hindered enone face opposite the methyl substituent at C4.[3] Thus, the diastereomer with the alkyl groups that are trans to each other predominates. If the starting material is racemic, an equal amount of the enantiomer will form, but the stereochemistry of the substituents relative to each other will remain the same. In the enantioselective reaction shown below,[4] the substrate is achiral, and the chiral catalyst that is formed by the interaction of the intermediate organocopper species and the chiral ligand dictates which face of the alkene is attacked. Because the competing diastereomeric transition states are of different energies, one product enantiomer is formed preferentially over its antipode.

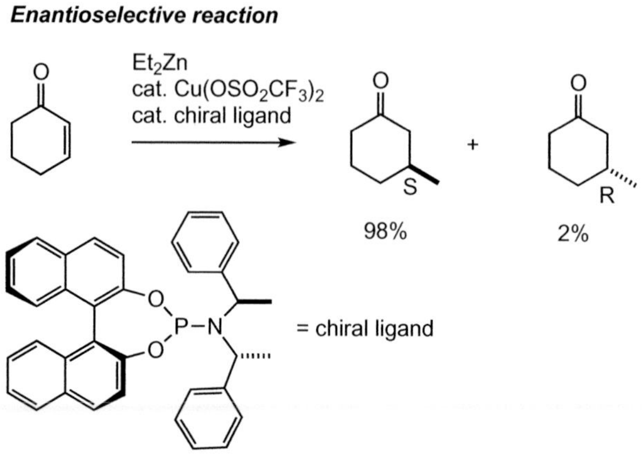

Enantioselective reaction

98%   2%

= chiral ligand

PROSPECTIVE SYNTHETIC PLANNING

Early synthetic efforts were typically prospective in nature. That is, one started with a readily available starting material and used reliable reactions to build up the structure until one reached the target. One of the pioneers of organic chemistry was Emil Fischer (1852–1919; developer of the Fischer projection, Fischer esterification, and the lock and key model for enzymatic action; winner of the 1902 Nobel Prize in Chemistry). His work to prepare and identify the stereoisomers of the monosaccharides is a classic example of prospective synthetic planning. The resulting Kiliani–Fischer monosaccharide synthesis (Figure 1.3) starts with D-glyceraldehyde and involves the repetitive application of two known reactions (1. cyanohydrin formation, 2. semi-hydrogenation of the nitrile followed by hydrolysis of the intermediate imine) to build a complex molecule from simpler precursors. Although not usually recognized, the planning of this synthesis must have involved some retrospective thinking as well because the homologated α-hydroxyaldehyde was "connected" to its precursor α-hydroxyaldehyde through a common cyanohydrin. However, there are limitations to this approach. The Kiliani–Fischer synthesis of D-glucose is relatively straightforward, as it involved the application of just two simple reactions, albeit in an iterative manner. Note that the hydrocyanation reaction produced two diastereomeric products, which had to be separated before proceeding. The situation becomes more complicated when the synthesis of a target molecule requires the introduction of diverse functionality as in the case of Nirmatrelvir. Where does one start? A new paradigm for planning a synthesis is needed.

MODERN APPROACHES TO SYNTHETIC PLANNING

Given its limitations, it is not surprising that the use of the prospective approach has been replaced by a systematic approach to planning a synthesis that begins with a retrospective analysis of the target's molecular structure. The four organic chemists shown below are considered by many as true masters in the field of organic

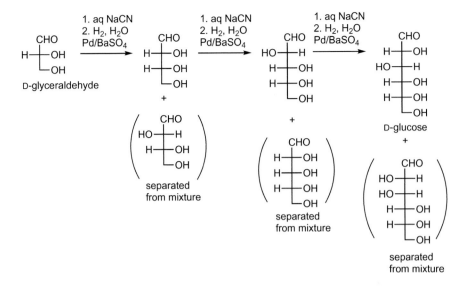

FIGURE 1.3. Kiliani–Fischer synthesis of D-glucose.

synthesis and have had a major impact on modern synthetic planning. They are Robert Robinson (1886–1975), R. B. Woodward (1917–1979), Gilbert Stork (1921–2017), and E. J. Corey (1928–). Robinson, Woodward, and Corey won Nobel Prizes in Chemistry for their contributions.

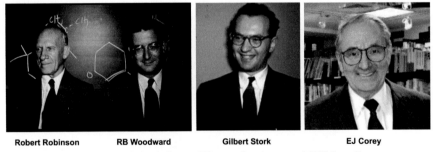

| Robert Robinson | RB Woodward | Gilbert Stork | EJ Corey |

Photos are courtesy of the Science History Institute and Wikimedia.

Robinson's synthesis of **tropinone** was a seminal event that laid the foundation for modern retrospective analysis and is a classic example of a natural product synthesis.[5] Tropinone is an alkaloid precursor of atropine, a compound used to treat organophosphate poisoning.

Robinson recognized that the tropinone structure contained two symmetrically arranged β-aminoketones, and he realized that these substructures could be created in a single reaction via a properly designed double Mannich reaction (Figure 1.4). This insight defined the disconnections that lead to the starting materials. The Robinson synthesis of tropinone involved an early example of what we will call

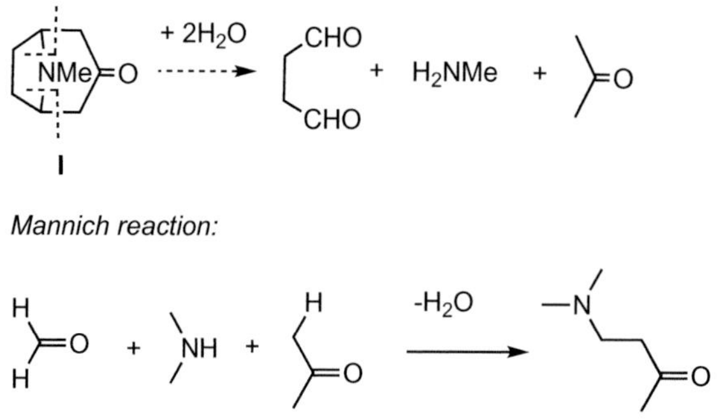

Mannich reaction:

FIGURE 1.4.   Robinson's "imaginary hydrolysis" of tropinone and the Mannich reaction.

"pattern recognition" later on in this chapter. His plan for the synthesis of tropinone is reproduced below, just as he described it in his original paper:

> *Nevertheless, an inspection of the formula of tropinone (I) discloses a degree of symmetry and an architecture which justify the hope that the base may ultimately be obtained in good yield as the product of some simple reaction and from accessible materials. By imaginary hydrolysis at the points indicated by the dotted lines, the substance may be resolved into succindialdehyde, methylamine, and acetone, and this observation suggested a line of attack of the problem which resulted in a direct synthesis.*

The tropinone plan involved the integration of both retrospective (pattern recognition and bond disconnections) and prospective (use of the Mannich reaction) thinking. This may well be a consequence of how the human brain is wired. By imagining the breaking of the indicted bonds, he likely had the Mannich reaction in mind. In practice, the actual synthesis (Figure 1.5) involved the use of an acetone surrogate, acetone dicarboxylate (acetone itself would have the propensity to self-condense), which undergoes a double decarboxylation after the double Mannich reaction. The yield of this multicomponent and "green" reaction is remarkable when one considers the side reactions that could compete with the desired sequence of events.[*]

Retrosynthetic analysis provides a highly organized conceptual framework for synthetic planning that involves the logical dismantling of a more complex molecule into simpler components via the stepwise disconnection of key bonds. This results in complementary reaction sequences, each of which could form the basis for a synthetic plan. Thus, the retrosynthetic analysis process may be viewed as the trading of

---

[*] However, innovation is not born in a vacuum! Apparently, Robinson was not the only person to perform this retrosynthetic disconnection of the tropinone molecule. Exactly how much other scientists influenced his thinking on this subject is a matter of speculation (Birch, A. J. (1993). Investigating a scientific legend: the tropinone synthesis of Sir Robert Robinson, FR S. *Notes and Records of the Royal Society of London*, 47(2), 277–296). One must note that it is extremely difficult to come up with a truly original idea. Regardless of how the ideas embodied in his synthesis of tropinone were actually formulated, it was Robinson who put the ideas into practice, and he deserves the credit that he has since received. In his own words: "Only results count."

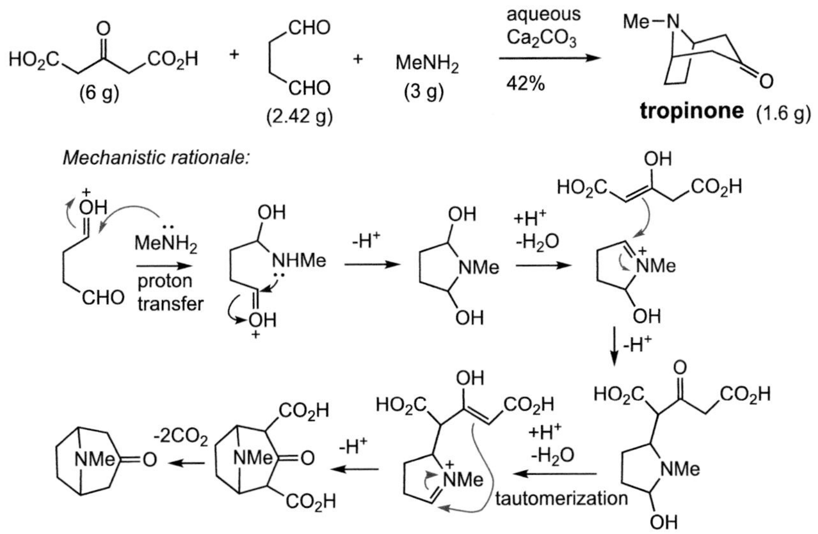

FIGURE 1.5. Robinson's one-pot synthesis of tropinone.

molecular complexity for synthetic options. Corey pioneered the use of retrosynthetic analysis and its application to synthetic planning.[6] To understand this concept, let us look at a five-reaction sequence used to synthesize a moth pheromone from the reverse direction (Figure 1.6). That is, let's view the sequence beginning with the final product and ending with the starting material. The forward synthetic reaction sequence is shown on the left. On the right, we show the corresponding retrosynthetic sequence. Note that a special arrow is used in the retrosynthetic complement to a reaction. The detailed reagents need not be provided at this stage of the analysis.

A **transform** describes the reverse of a chemical reaction in which the product is transformed into the starting molecule. A **retron** is the minimal molecular subunit in the product that "actuates" a specific transform. In this scheme, the acetate ester is the retron for the first transform, the primary alcohol is the retron for the second transform, the trans alkene is the retron for the third transform, and the alkylated alkyne is the retron for the fourth and fifth transforms.

For complex molecules, more than one retron is usually present, and this results in the branching of the retrosynthetic paths. This branching leads to what is known colloquially as an **inverted synthesis tree** (Figure 1.7). One can then evaluate the branches for feasibility and "prune" the tree.

Corey formalized a series of **retrosynthetic strategies**. The application of these analysis tools results in the generation of multiple paths that comprise the inverted synthesis tree. For any given synthesis, multiple strategies may be (and usually are) employed during the analysis phase:

- Transform-based strategies: identify a key transform that rapidly reduces molecular complexity. If necessary, functionality may be added to the structure to create a retron.

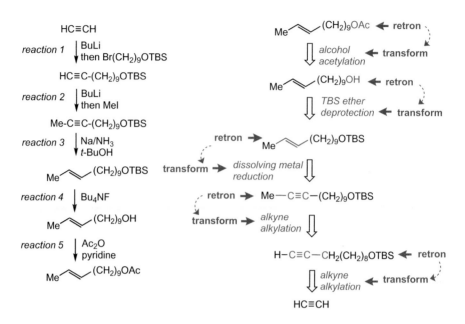

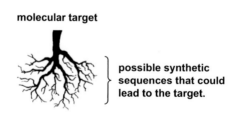

FIGURE 1.6. A five-reaction synthetic sequence (left) compared with its corresponding retrosynthetic transform sequence (right). The connection between the retrons and their transforms are shown in red.

- Structure-based strategies: identify a key structural unit that maps onto a readily available starting material. This is particularly valuable when stereochemistry is involved.
- Topological strategies: identify key bonds to break in a retrosynthetic analysis. Retron functionality can be added if needed. It is very useful when multiple rings are fused together.
- Stereochemical strategies: attempt to identify retrons that generate stereocenters present in the target molecule during C–C bond-forming reactions.
- Descriptions of these retrosynthetic strategies along with examples of their use follows.
- **Transform-based strategies** begin with the identification of a key transform or tactical combination of transforms. This is probably the strategy that is used most often in combination with the next three strategies. *Let's consider the following examples.*

molecular target

possible synthetic sequences that could lead to the target.

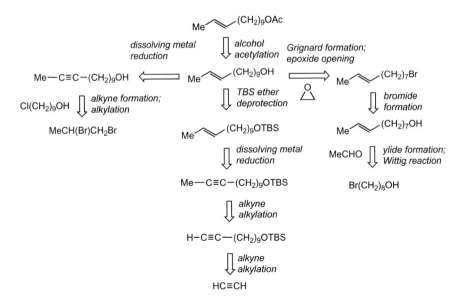

FIGURE 1.7. An inverted synthesis tree.

THE ROBINSON ANNULATION TRANSFORM

An example[7] of the Robinson annulation in action, along with its overall mechanism, is shown in Figure 1.8. This annulation (ring formation) proceeds in two stages, the first being a Michael reaction and the second being an aldol condensation. Although alternative aldol closures are possible, the one that is shown is favored because it alone can form a stable enone. The product is known as the Wieland-Miescher ketone, which is a starting material used in many syntheses.

*In Figure 1.9, we show the same Robinson annulation in its reverse format, as would be seen in a retrosynthetic analysis. The magenta colored cyclohexenone substructure is the retron for this **powerful transform**. A transform may be considered "powerful" if it involves the disconnection of two or more skeletal bonds. Because the Robinson annulation involves the tactical combinatiom of two transforms with the latter dependent on the former, it could also be described as a nested transform.*

Sometimes a retron is "hidden" and must be found. In such cases, it may be necessary to add functionality to a molecule to create a retron. This may seem to be counterintuitive, as it entails adding functionality rather than removing it. However, this can often be justified if the modification reveals a powerful transform. In the second example, a double bond is added (hydrogenation transform) to the target molecule generating the Robinson annulation retron.

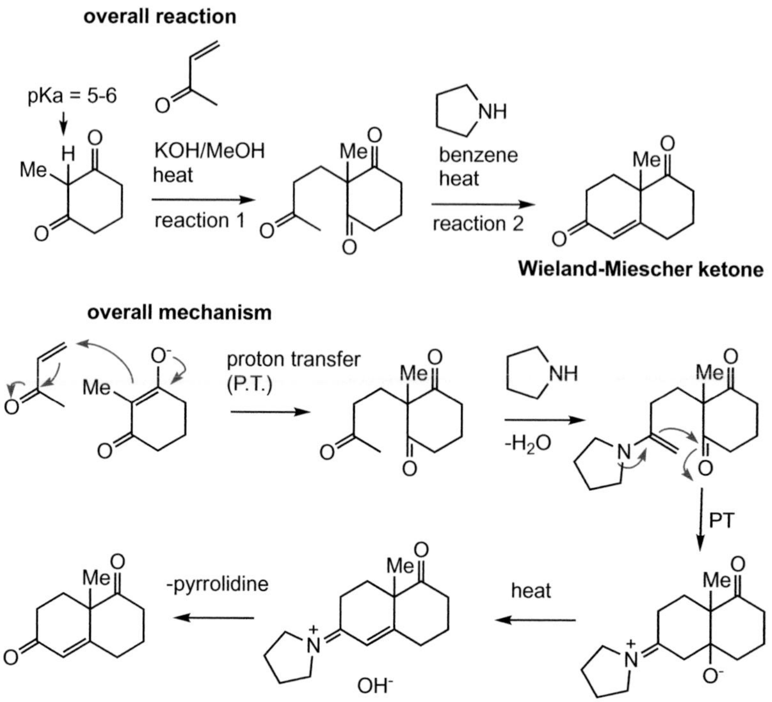

overall reaction

Wieland-Miescher ketone

overall mechanism

FIGURE 1.8.   An example of the Robinson annulation and its mechanism.

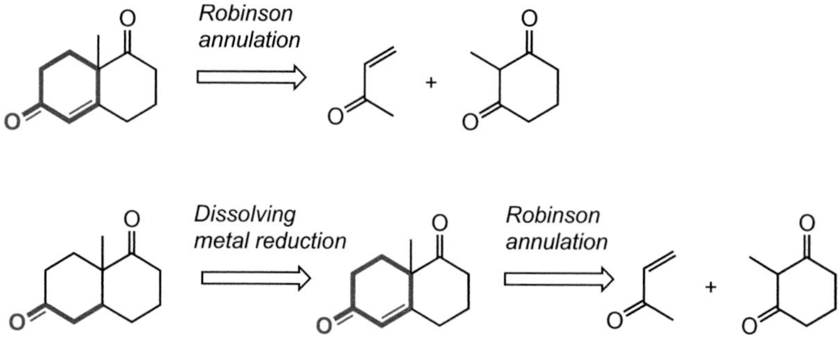

FIGURE 1.9.   Obvious and hidden Robinson annulation transforms. Retrons are magenta.

The recognition of retrons in complex molecules can reveal powerful transforms that greatly simplify the synthesis. Consider the key step in Majetich's synthesis of perovskone (Figure 1.10).[8] In this single reaction, five skeletal bonds, six stereocenters, and four rings are created. A retrosynthetic breakdown of the individual steps in this reaction is shown in Figure 1.11. Identification of the Diels–Alder retron in

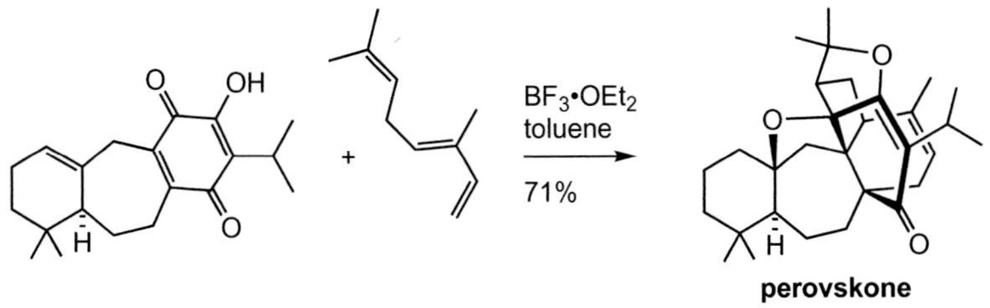

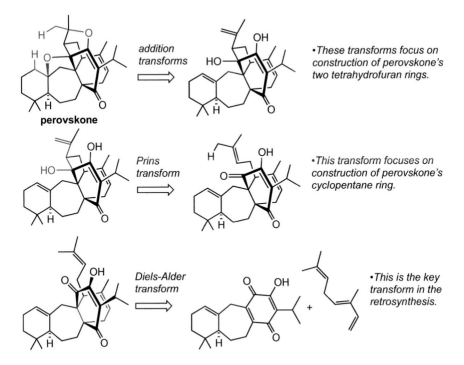

FIGURE 1.10. Key step in Majetich's synthesis of perovskone.

*the structure (the magenta-colored cyclohexene ring) enabled the application of this powerful transform. Careful analysis of the structural relationship between perovs-kone and the Diels–Alder product reveals two additional transforms: an intramo-lecular Prins reaction and two intramolecular Markovnikov additions of an alcohol across two trisubstituted alkenes. Together, the three transforms form a **reaction cascade** or what may be considered a **"nested" transform**. That is, they each create the retron that enables the subsequent transform. Because all three reactions are catalyzed by acid, the entire sequence occurs in one reaction vessel, which makes the synthesis particularly efficient and green.*

addition transforms

• These transforms focus on construction of perovskone's two tetrahydrofuran rings.

perovskone

Prins transform

• This transform focuses on construction of perovskone's cyclopentane ring.

Diels-Alder transform

• This is the key transform in the retrosynthesis.

FIGURE 1.11. The perovskone reaction cascade and the concept of "nested" transforms.

Forward reaction

Me—Me $\overset{+}{\text{C}}$ R + R'$\overset{\overset{\text{OBF}_3}{}}{\underset{}{}}$R" $\xrightarrow{\text{Lewis or}\atop\text{Brönsted acid}}$ Me OBF$_3$ ... R" $\xrightarrow{\text{proton}\atop\text{transfer}\atop -\text{BF}_3}$ Me R' R" OH

Retrosynthetic transform

Me R' R" ... OH $\overset{\textit{Prins}}{\underset{\textit{transform}}{\Longrightarrow}}$ Me—Me R + R'$\overset{O}{\underset{}{}}$R"

FIGURE 1.12.   The Prins reaction with its retron colored magenta.

This is likely your first exposure to the Prins reaction. A general description of the variant used in the perovskone synthesis is shown in Figure 1.12. This reaction proceeds through a carbenium ion (a trivalent carbocation) intermediate, followed by elimination, and ultimately results in the formation of a homoallylic alcohol. A number of synthetically useful variations exist for the Prins reaction that depend on the structure of the substrate, but they all involve the formation of a carbenium ion intermediate.[9]

The process of identifying retrons that are embedded in complex molecular structures, such as perovskone, involves **pattern recognition**.[10] *This can be quite challenging when the retron consists of multiple transforms that are linked together (as in the perovskone example), but the human brain has evolved so that—with a little practice—we can learn to recognize these visual patterns.*

If you've ever hunted for morels (a type of spring mushroom) in the forest, you might pass by specimens because you don't recognize the morel's pattern. But once you find your first morel, the pattern becomes engraved in your memory, and it is much easier to find the next one. (Pattern recognition is also necessary to distinguish between true morels and poisonous false morels.) Thus, practice makes it easier! The same goes for molecular pattern recognition.

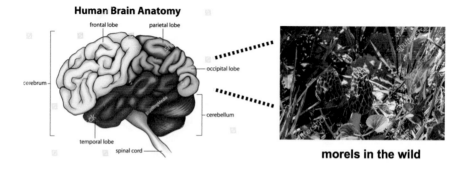

morels in the wild

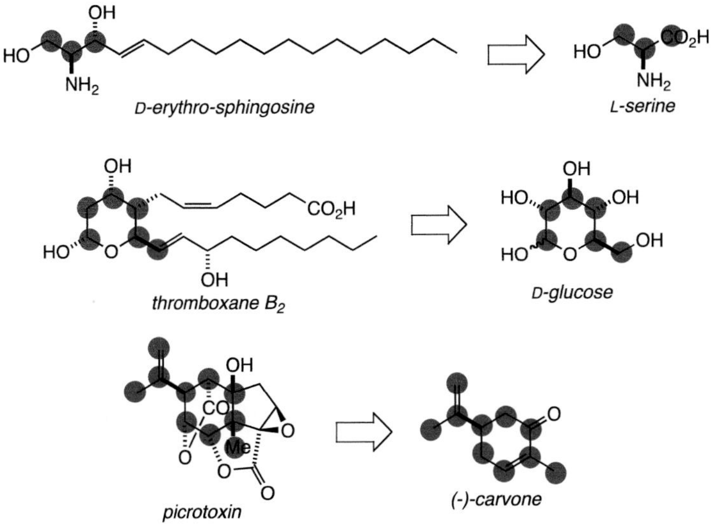

FIGURE 1.13. Examples of structure-based strategies. The product carbon atoms that are derived from the starting material are highlighted in magenta.

Structure-based strategies involve the identification of a potential starting material, building block, retrosynthetic subunit, or initiating element that leads to major simplification.

In these three examples (Figure 1.13), one can easily identify the carbon backbones of serine, glucose, and carvone in the targets' structures (highlighted in magenta). However, the use of a readily available starting material does not necessarily guarantee the most step-efficient synthesis, as additional functionality may need to be removed, modified, and/or added.

Topological strategies involve the reduction of molecular connectivity through the application of rules that guide the selection of bonds for disconnection.

FOR ACYCLIC SYSTEMS, THESE RULES ARE

- *Preserve building block or structure goal entities.*
- *Disconnect to structures of nearly equal complexity.*
- *Disconnect C-X (heteroatom) or internal C=C bonds.*
- *Disconnect up to three bonds from functional groups.*
- *Disconnect to reduce the number of stereocenters.*

FOR FUSED, BRIDGED, AND SPIRO RING SYSTEMS, ADD

- *Disconnect primary (usually 5- or 6-membered) ring bonds.*
- *Disconnect ring bonds to reduce bridging.*

Consider the following plan for the synthesis of the pheromone of the beetle that causes Dutch elm disease. The application of the first five topological rules for acyclic systems identifies the optimal retrosynthetic disconnection as the C3–C4 bond.

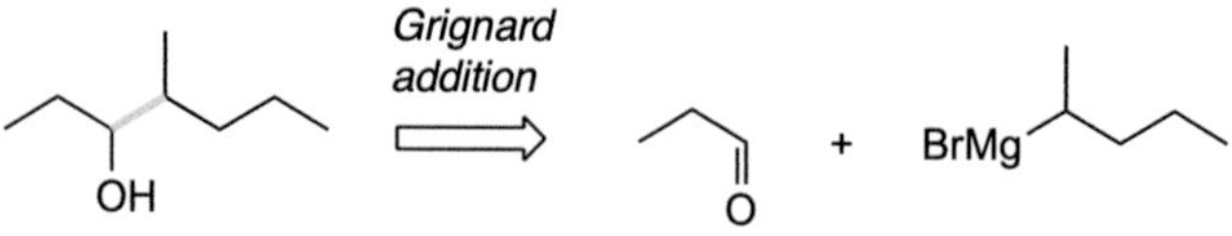

However, if one starts out with a ketone reduction transform, an enolate alkylation transform is revealed enabling disconnection at the C4–C5 bond.

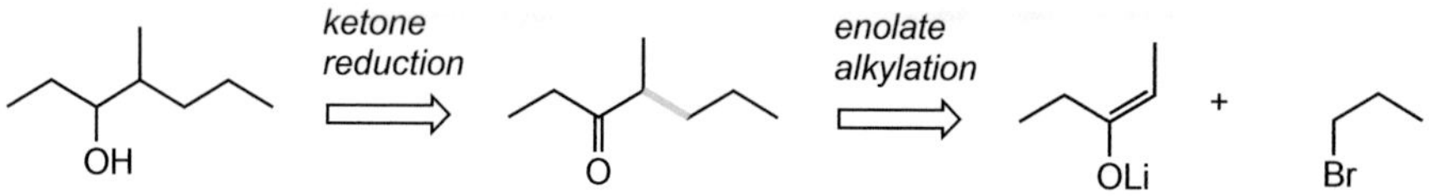

In this second case, we needed to change one functional group (2°alcohol) into another (ketone) to obtain the key C–C bond-breaking enolate alkylation retron. Note that we have been ignoring the issue of stereochemistry at this level of analysis. In the end, both disconnections are reasonable. The choice of which path to follow might depend on the availability and/or cost of the starting materials and reagents involved.

In devising a synthesis of the sesquiterpene natural product longifolene,[11] application of the topological strategy rules identifies the best bond to break but does not reveal a viable retron. Modification of the target structure is required to install a 1,5-diketone substructure, which is the retron for a Michael addition. Thus, it can be seen that a mixture of strategies was used to arrive at a viable synthetic plan.

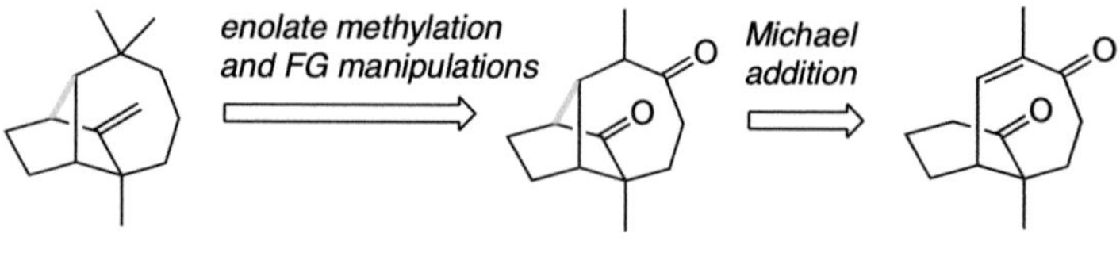

One need not define the exact reaction conditions at this level of the analysis. The details of the reaction to be performed in the synthesis can be added later, often with the help of a program such as SciFinder or Reaxys. In Corey's synthesis of longifolene, the key Michael addition was accomplished as follows:

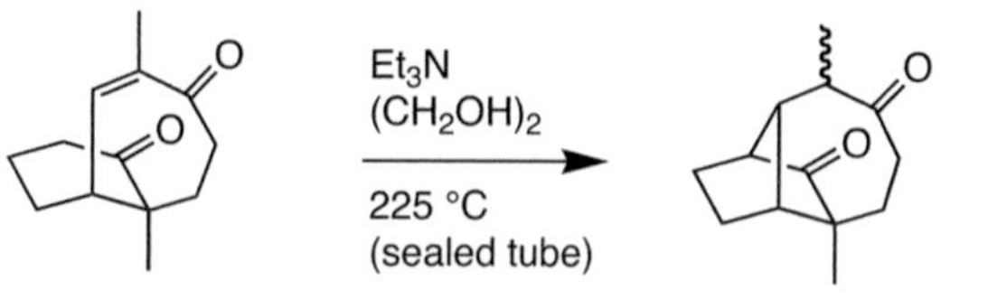

Stereochemical strategies endeavor to reduce molecular complexity through the retrosynthetic elimination of stereocenters.

In the first example, three stereocenters in the target can be eliminated by application of an enolate alkylation transform because the starting ketone has a plane of symmetry and is achiral. The alkylation would be selective for the (racemic) diastereomer shown due to the cup-like shape of the molecule. In the second example, three chiral centers are generated in an intermolecular Diels–Alder reaction between an achiral diene and an achiral dienophile. An endo transition state is preferred because of secondary orbital overlap, so the endo diastereomer predominates.

A WORD ABOUT SYNTHETIC EFFICIENCY

The most attractive syntheses are efficient. The simplest metric for judging the overall efficiency is the number of steps in the longest linear sequence of reactions. Gaich and Baran have carried the evaluation of efficiency further by defining the ideal synthesis:[12]

$$\% \text{ideality} = \frac{(\text{construction rxns} + \text{strategic redox rxns}) \times 100}{(\text{total no. of steps})}$$

- **Construction reactions** form skeletal bonds (C–C and C–heteroatom).
- **Strategic redox reactions** directly establish the correct functionality found in the final product.

All other reactions are viewed as "concession steps." For example, the use of a protecting group usually adds concession steps to the reaction sequence. Analysis of the five-step synthesis of the moth pheromone (Figure 1.6) reveals that Steps 1, 2, 3, and 5 are construction steps, while Step 4 is a concession step making the synthesis 80% ideal.

We suggest a modification to the equation that recognizes the use of reactions that form multiple skeletal bonds (cycloadditions, domino reactions) by adding "1" to the numerator for each additional bond formed in a reaction. For example, a sequence that includes a Diels–Alder reaction (2 skeletal bonds formed) would add "1" to the numerator.

$$\% \text{ideality} = \frac{\left(\begin{array}{c} \text{construction} \\ \text{reactions} \end{array} + \begin{array}{c} \text{strategic} \\ \text{redox reactions} \end{array} + \begin{array}{c} \text{multi} - \text{bond} \\ \text{bonus} \end{array}\right)}{(\text{total reactions})} \times 100$$

A WORD ABOUT PROTECTING GROUPS

The inherent inefficiency associated with the use of a protecting group can be minimized if the protecting group itself is part of the target structure. If multiple protecting groups are involved, the number of concession steps can be reduced if the deprotections can be performed with a single reagent. The liability associated with the use of a protecting group can also be mitigated if the protecting group plays an additional role in the synthesis such as controlling stereochemistry or altering solubility.

A WORD ABOUT THE USE OF CHEMICAL DATABASES

Chemical databases such as SciFinder and Reaxys are powerful computer-based tools that can be very useful for designing a synthetic plan. They may also have a limited capability to perform retrosynthetic analyses using the target structure as input. In our opinion, the primary value of such programs lies in the ability to search the chemical literature for specific molecular structures and reactions. However, such programs are especially powerful when used as an adjunct to the organic chemist's own intuition. We find these databases particularly useful for defining experimental conditions and finding known reactions when you follow the planning protocol that is described below.

TUTORIAL: THE HOLISTIC APPROACH ILLUSTRATED—PLANNING A
SYNTHESIS OF THE BICYCLIC AMINO ACID COMPONENT OF PAXLOVID

1. **Identify functional groups in the target molecule noting whether they activate proximal carbon atoms.**

Nirmatrelvir contains four amides: a nitrile, a cyclopropane, a pyrrolidine, and a pyrrolidone moiety. The carbons that are alpha to the amide carbonyl are activated and can stabilize an anion or, in certain situations, a radical. The methylene carbon alpha to the pyrrolidine nitrogen can stabilize a carbocation or radical.

2. **Identify patterns that employ powerful transforms or readily available starting materials. If necessary, add functional groups to create powerful retrons.**

The amide bonds, which are the formal result of condensation between a carboxylic acid and an amine, may be subjected to imaginary hydrolysis to give the three unnatural amino acids shown below. The compound on the far left has an unprotected carboxylic acid, while the compound on the far right has an unprotected amine. However, the presence of both functional groups in the central bicyclic amino acid will require the use of a protecting group to ensure chemoselectivity during peptide bond formation.

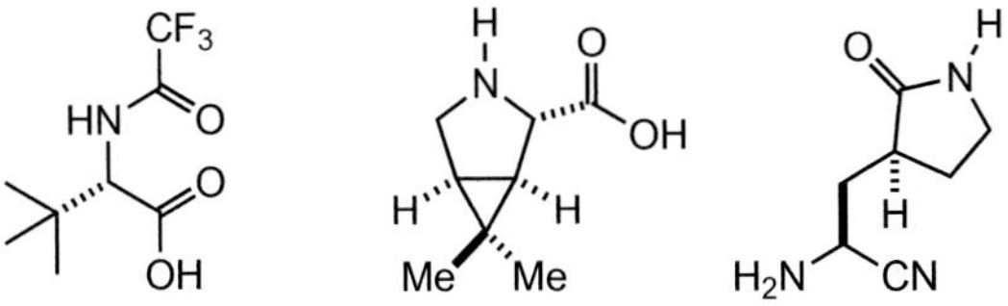

Focusing on the synthesis of the bicyclic amino acid component (the middle compound), we note that the cyclopropane and pyrrolidine rings are retrons for cycloaddition transforms that generate two C–C bonds in one step via carbenes (Path A) and azomethine ylides (Path B), respectively. A third strategy will involve the conversion of a readily available commodity chemical to the target.

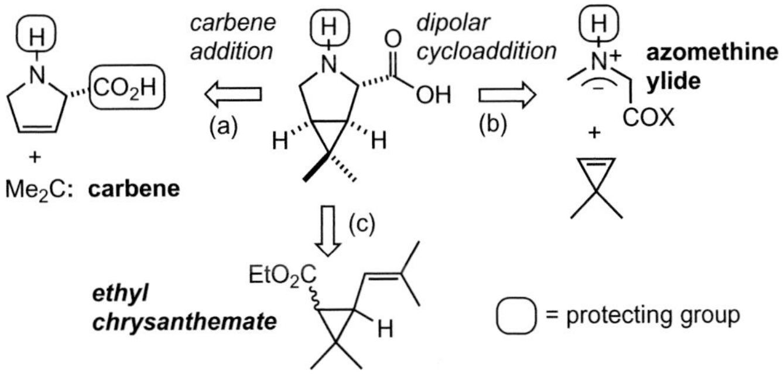

CARBENES AND CARBENOIDS

Carbenes are reactive divalent carbon species that can add to double and triple bonds to form cyclopropanes and cyclopropenes, respectively. They can also insert into single bonds. Free carbenes are electron-deficient because they only have six valence electrons. Carbenes may also coordinate to metals, in which case they are described as carbenoids. A convenient way to access synthetically useful carbenes involves exposing a geminal dibromide to n-BuLi. If this reaction is performed in the presence of an alkene, a cyclopropane will form. However, there will be a problem applying this reaction to the unsaturated proline because the strongly nucleophilic n-BuLi will undoubtedly react with the carbonyl-based protecting groups. A milder reagent is needed. It turns out that n-BuLi can be replaced by zinc metal (the Simmons–Smith reaction)[14] or diethylzinc (the Furukawa variant thereof), resulting in an organometallic intermediate capable of formally adding a carbene across a double bond. The formal addition of dimethyl carbene to (E)-alkenes produces trans-disubstituted cyclopropanes, whereas the addition to a (Z)-alkene produces cis-disubstituted alkenes. An even more effective reaction results if a cobaltc(II)-based catalyst is added, enabling the use of geminal dichlorides as carbene precursors. These Simmons–Smith variants tolerate a wide range of functional groups.

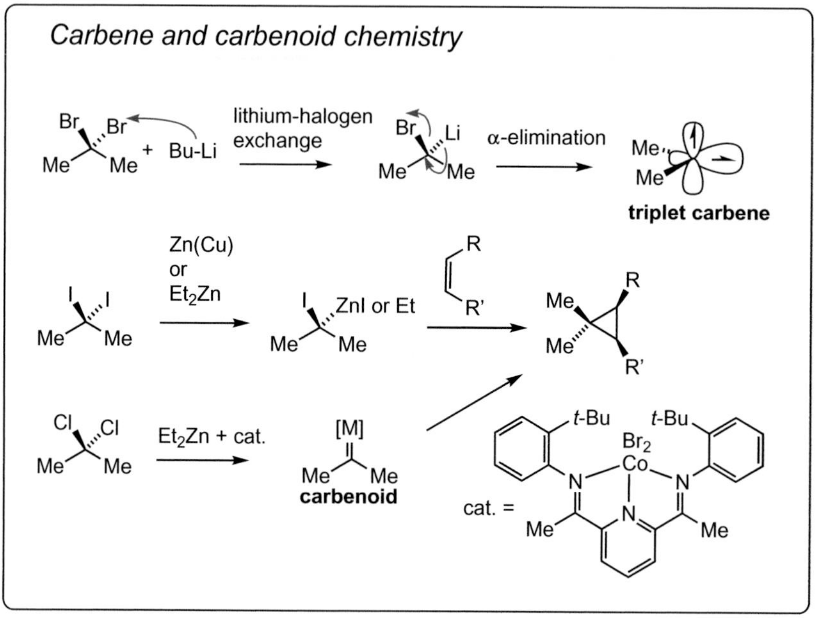

AZOMETHINE YLIDES

Azomethine ylides are reactive species (neutral dipoles) that cycloadd to alkenes to give pyrrolidines. Pyrrolidines are ubiquitous motifs in alkaloid natural products and drugs. A comparison between the frontier molecular orbital interactions in the Diels–Alder and azomethine ylide cycloadditions is shown below.[13] The azomethine ylide is a molecular construct that you may not be familiar with. However, it is related to the Diels–Alder diene that you should be familiar with. Like Diels–Alder dienes, azomethine ylides contain 4π electrons, but they are distributed between three sp²-hybridized atoms rather than four atoms. Dienes undergo suprafacial cycloaddition with dienophiles to give cyclohexenes, while azomethines ylides undergo suprafacial dipolar cycloaddition with dipolarophiles to give pyrrolidines.

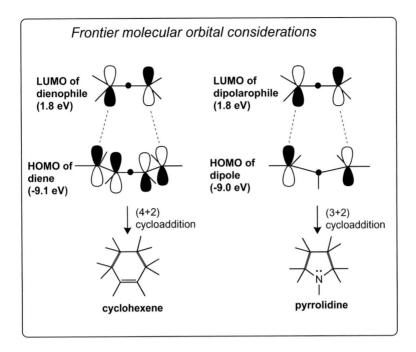

The rate of the cycloaddition reaction can be increased by reducing the frontier HOMO–LUMO energy gap. This is usually done by placing electron withdrawing substituents on the dienophile and dipolarophile, thus lowering the LUMO energy. The activation barrier can also be lowered by making the reaction unimolecular, connecting the two components via a molecular tether. Azomethine ylides may be chiral by virtue of their permanent substituents, removable chiral auxiliaries, or their interaction with chiral catalysts, leading to asymmetric cycloadditions.

3. **Continue your analysis until you reach readily available starting materials.**

(Path A) Starting with the monoprotected bicyclic amino acid, the first transform involves deprotection of the carboxylic acid. The second transform installs the cyclopropane ring via carbene addition to the 3,4-dehydroproline (**transform-based and stereochemical strategies**). The carbenoid is expected to add to the alkene face opposite the protected carboxylic acid because of its steric bulk. The unsaturated pyrrolidine is formed by the net dehydration of 4-hydroxyproline. The final two transforms are concerned with protection of the amine and carboxylic acid functional groups. The starting material, trans-4-hydroxyproline is a constituent of collagen and is readily available as a byproduct of bovine and porcine processing (**structure-based strategy**).

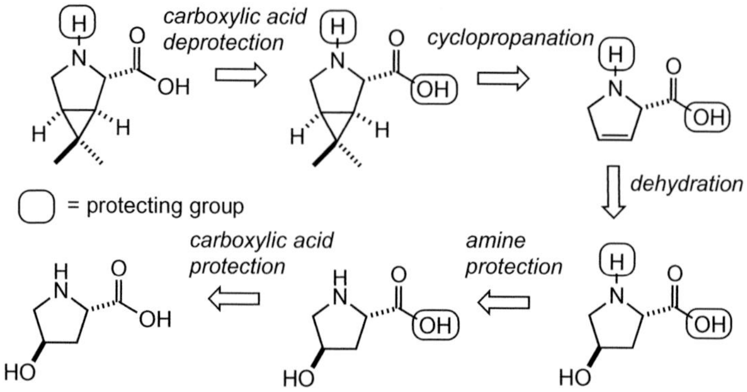

= protecting group

4. Write out a synthetic plan that includes the reagents that will be used for each reaction.

The synthetic plan begins with protection of the carboxylic acid and amine. The hydroxyl group is then activated by conversion to a triflate that undergoes a base-induced elimination to give the 3-alkene. It is possible that competing elimination will give the 4-alkene as well, but we won't be concerned with this potential problem at this level of analysis. A dimethylcarbene or carbenoid will be added to the double bond on its β-face. Saponification of the methyl ester produces the carboxylic acid that is ready to couple to a primary amine.

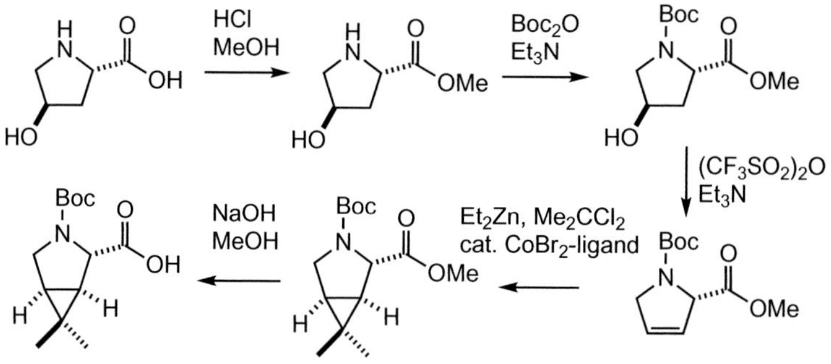

5. To compare alternate paths, repeat Steps 1 through 4 making different disconnections until reaching readily available starting materials.

An alternative plan (Path B) employs a chiral auxiliary (X*) to set the developing stereochemistry. Chiral auxiliaries function by converting enantiomeric transition states of the same energy into diastereomeric transition states that have different energies. Because of this difference, the reaction pathway with the lowest activation energy will be favored, resulting in the preferential formation of one diastereomer.

Removal of the chiral auxiliary converts the diastereomer into an enantiomer, thus making the net process enantioselective. The key transform involves an asymmetric dipolar cycloaddition of a chiral azomethine ylide and 3,3-dimethyl cyclopropene (**stereochemical and transform-based strategies**). *The reactive azomethine ylide is formed by heating a precursor aziridine to initiate electrocyclic conrotatory ring opening (analogous to cyclobutene opening to 1,3-butadiene). The azomethine ylide undergoes concerted suprafacial addition to the cyclopropene, which is expected to be activated by ring strain. Support for this expectation comes from the fact that 3,3-dimethylcyclopropene is known to undergo Diels–Alder reactions with 1,3-dienes.*

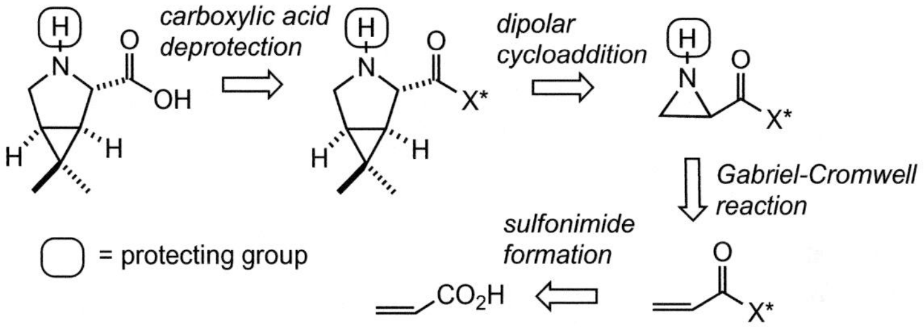

The aziridine is readily prepared by a Gabriel–Cromwell reaction sequence that involves the addition of bromine to an α,β -unsaturated carbonyl compound followed by elimination of HBr to give α -bromo substituted system. An amine then adds to the β -carbon and, after auxiliary-controlled protonation of the enolate, displaces the α -bromine atom to form the enantiopure aziridine.

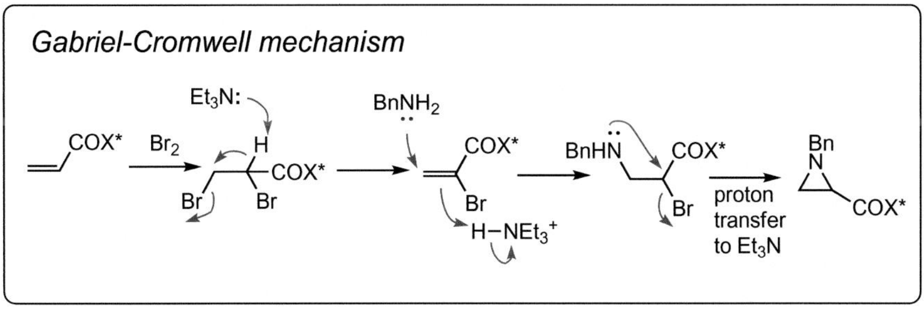

In the synthetic direction, we begin with the Gabriel–Cromwell reaction, which provides convenient access to the aziridine. The chiral auxiliary (X*) is known as Oppolzer's camphorsultam and is derived from camphor, a naturally occurring terpene. Heating the chiral aziridine in the presence of 3,3-dimethylcyclopropene will result in a concerted electrocyclic ring opening to a chiral azomethine ylide[15] that cycloadds to the cyclopropane to give a bicyclic pyrrolidine.

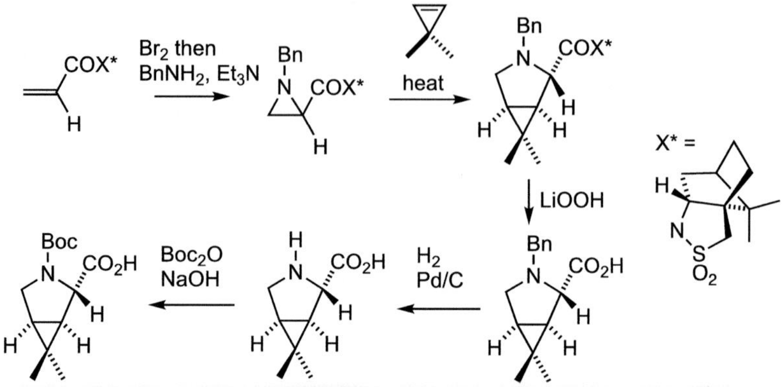

COX* — Br₂ then BnNH₂, Et₃N → Bn N COX* — heat → Bn N COX*

$X^* =$

↓ LiOOH

Boc N CO₂H ← Boc₂O NaOH — H N CO₂H ← H₂ Pd/C — Bn N CO₂H

A third option (Path C) may also be envisioned that begins with an intramolecular application of the Strecker amino acid synthesis with the iminium ion (a ring-chain tautomer of an aminoaldehyde) derived from an azido aldehyde. This aldehyde is obtained by ozonolysis of the trisubstituted double bond. The azide is formed by displacement of a mesylate that is derived from cis-chrysanthemol. This alcohol is produced by the reduction of the corresponding ethyl ester generated from a commercially available mixture of racemic cis- and trans-ethyl chrysanthemate.

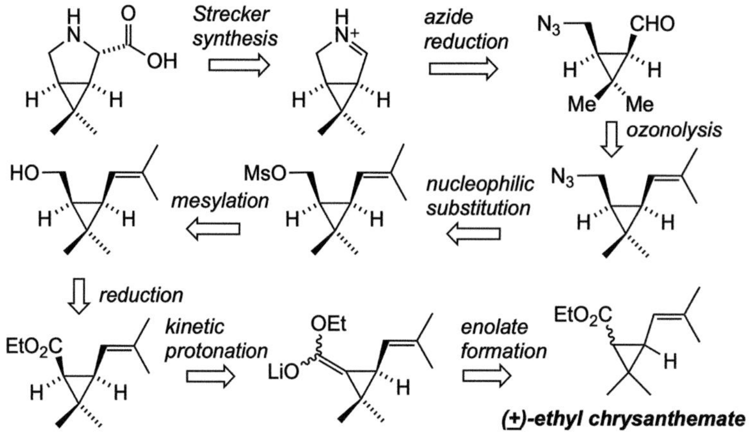

Strecker synthesis ⟹

azide reduction ⟹

ozonolysis ⟹

mesylation ⟸

nucleophilic substitution ⟸

reduction ⇓

kinetic protonation ⟹

enolate formation ⟹

(±)-ethyl chrysanthemate

In the forward direction, the synthetic sequence involves enolate formation at low temperature using lithium diisopropylamide (LDA) as the base. Protonation will preferentially take place on the least hindered face of the enolate and if conducted in an aprotic solvent at low temperature, produce the less stable cis-configured product under irreversible conditions. The Strecker addition of cyanide to the convex face of an iminium ion intermediate (not shown) will produce the desired relative stereochemistry, providing another option for adjustment of the relative stereochemistry. There are no obvious chemistry problems to be noted. However, the sequence produces racemic material, necessitating a resolution if enantiomerically pure product is desired.

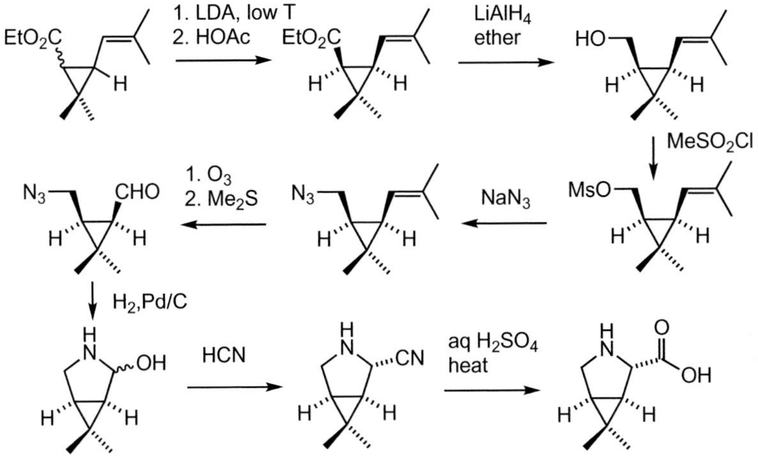

STEREOCONTROL CONSIDERATIONS

The stereochemical outcome of the azomethine ylide cycloaddition in Path B depends on the conformational preference of the azomethine ylide. Literature precedents[15] suggest that the camphorsultam auxiliary developed by Oppolzer will adopt a conformation that minimizes the net dipole by placing the carbonyl and sulfur dioxide moieties "anti" to each other. From X-ray studies, we know that the nitrogen atom in such compounds is slightly pyramidalized. This places the pro-S oxygen atom (colored red) closer to the α -carbon, blocking the reapproach of the dipolarphile. The author of this primer is familiar with the use of Oppolzer's auxiliary to control developing stereocenters in dipolar cycloadditions because of work that was performed in his laboratory. However, if one didn't have such knowledge, the generic representation of a chiral auxiliary (X) would be satisfactory for an initial retrosynthetic plan with the understanding that a suitable chiral auxiliary exists and could be found. There are two places in Path C where the relative stereochemistry can be adjusted. The first option involves the kinetic (irreversible) protonation of the enolate derived from the starting ester, and the second is the Strecker reaction during the cyanide addition to the iminium ion.*

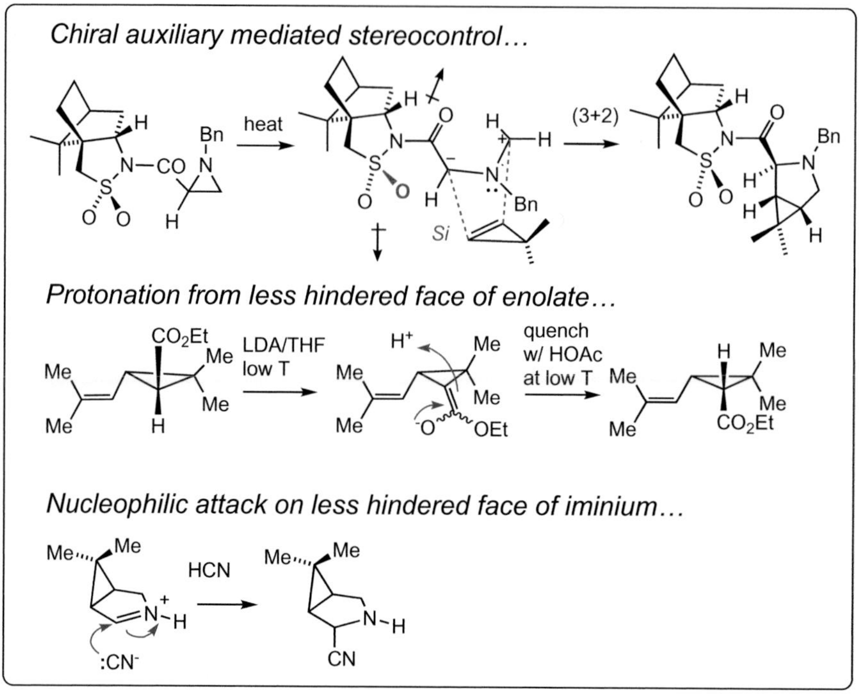

Chiral auxiliary mediated stereocontrol...
heat
(3+2)
Bn
Si
Protonation from less hindered face of enolate...
LDA/THF
low T
quench
w/ HOAc
at low T
Nucleophilic attack on less hindered face of iminium...
HCN
:CN-

6. **Analyze each of the branches in terms of feasibility, rejecting branches that have major problems. If you have more than one viable branch, prioritize them.**

Path A consists of five steps, two of which are construction steps, and includes a reaction that makes two C–C bonds (add "1" to the numerator of the ideality equation), leading to a 60% ideality score. The product will be enantiomerically pure because it starts out with an enantiomerically pure amino acid. It is possible that the elimination reaction will produce a mixture of isomeric alkenes. Path B consists of five steps, two of which are construction steps, and includes a reaction that makes two C–C bonds (add "1" to the numerator of the ideality equation), leading to a 50% ideality score. There is a good chance that the product will be enantiomerically pure, though this depends on the diastereoselectivity of the azomethine ylide cycloaddition. Path C consists of eight steps, two of which are construction steps, leading to a 25% ideality score. Because this synthesis would produce racemic material, a resolution is required to obtain enantiomerically pure material. Based on these considerations, Paths A or B should be followed first.

SUMMARY

In this chapter, we proposed a rationale for the study of synthesis. We illustrate our thesis with a real-life application to the COVID-19 pandemic. Some thoughts on the impact that artificial intelligence has had (and will have) on synthetic planning was presented. This was followed by a review of basic concepts and a historical overview of how synthetic planning has evolved over the years. The role of pattern recognition in synthetic planning was illustrated as was the value of maintaining a well-stocked reaction "toolbox." Toward this end, the Robinson annulation mechanism, the relationship between the Diels–Alder and azomethine cycloadditions, carbene, and carbenoid-mediated cyclopropanations; the Prins reaction; and the Gabriel–Cromwell synthesis of aziridines were discussed. The use of chiral auxiliaries to control stereochemistry was introduced. Retrosynthetic analysis was illustrated and incorporated into a general six-step "holistic" protocol for planning the synthesis of an organic molecule. A simple qualitative approach for the evaluation of the efficiency of any given synthetic sequence was presented. The chapter concluded with a detailed example showing how this protocol can be applied to the synthesis of a key component of the COVID-19 antiviral Paxlovid.

REFERENCES

1. Owen, D. R., Allerton, C. M., Anderson, A. S., Aschenbrenner, L., Avery, M., Berritt, S., ... Zhu, Y. (2021). An oral SARS-CoV-2 Mpro inhibitor clinical candidate for the treatment of COVID-19. *Science, 374*(6575), 1586–1593.
2. Brown, H. C., & Zweifel, G. (1961). Hydroboration. IX. The hydroboration of cyclic and bicyclic olefins—Stereochemistry of the hydroboration reaction. *Journal of the American Chemical Society, 83*(11), 2544–2551.
3. Ouannes, C., Dressaire, G., & Langlois, Y. (1977). Influence de complexant sur la reactivite des organocuprates. *Tetrahedron Letters, 18*(10), 815–818.
4. López, F., Minnaard, A. J., & Feringa, B. L. (2007). Catalytic enantioselective conjugate addition with Grignard reagents. *Accounts of Chemical Research, 40*(3), 179–188.
5. Robinson, R. (1917). LXIII.—A synthesis of tropinone. *Journal of the Chemical Society, Transactions, 111*, 762–768.
6. Corey, E. J. (1991). The logic of chemical synthesis: Multistep synthesis of complex carbogenic molecules (Nobel lecture). *Angewandte Chemie International Edition in English, 30*(5), 455–465.
7. Ramachandran, S., & Newman, M. S. (2003). 1, 6-Dioxo-8a-Methyl-1, 2, 3, 4, 6, 7, 8, 8a-Octahydronaphthalene: 1, 6-Naphthalenedione, 1, 2, 3, 4, 6, 7, 8, 8a-octahydro-8a-methyl-. *Organic Syntheses, 41*, 38–38.
8. Majetich, G., Zhang, Y., Tian, X., Britton, J. E., Li, Y., & Phillips, R. (2011). Synthesis of (±)-and (+)-perovskone. *Tetrahedron, 67*(52), 10129–10146.
9. Doro, F., Akeroyd, N., Schiet, F., & Narula, A. (2019). The Prins reaction in the fragrance industry: 100th anniversary (1919–2019). *Angewandte Chemie, 131*(22), 7248–7253.
10. Wilson, R. M., & Danishefsky, S. J. (2007). Pattern recognition in retrosynthetic analysis: Snapshots in total synthesis. *The Journal of Organic Chemistry, 72*(12), 4293–4305.
11. Corey, E. J., Ohno, M., Mitra, R. B., & Vatakencherry, P. A. (1964). Total synthesis of longifolene. *Journal of the American Chemical Society, 86*(3), 478–485.
12. Gaich, T., & Baran, P. S. (2010). Aiming for the ideal synthesis. *The Journal of Organic Chemistry, 75*(14), 4657–4673.
13. Fleming, I. (2015). *Pericyclic reactions.* Oxford University Press. (A good primer that explains the role of molecular orbitals in Diels-Alder and dipolar cycloadditions as well as other pericyclic reactions.)

14. Charette, A. B., & Beauchemin, A. (2004). Simmons-smith cyclopropanation reaction. *Organic Reactions*, *58*, 1–415.
15. Garner, P., Dogan, Ö., Youngs, W. J., Kennedy, V. O., Protasiewicz, J., & Zaniewski, R. (2001). Stereocontrolled 1,3-dipolar cycloadditions using Oppolzer's camphor sultam as the chiral auxiliary for carbonyl stabilized azomethine ylides. *Tetrahedron*, *57*(1), 71–85.

PRACTICE PROBLEMS

1. Design a racemic synthesis of multistriatin following the holistic planning protocol, describing each step in detail. Note the retrosynthetic strategies that you used as well as any potential problems that you recognize. Label the retrons and write out the associated transforms. Determine the ideality of your synthesis. If you come up with multiple branches, prioritize them.

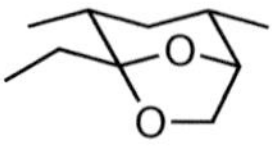

multistriatin

2. Find the hidden Diels–Alder reactions in the following structures. Circle the retron and show the diene and dienophile components. Will the cyclo-addition be facile? That is, are the components appropriately activated? Explain your reasoning.

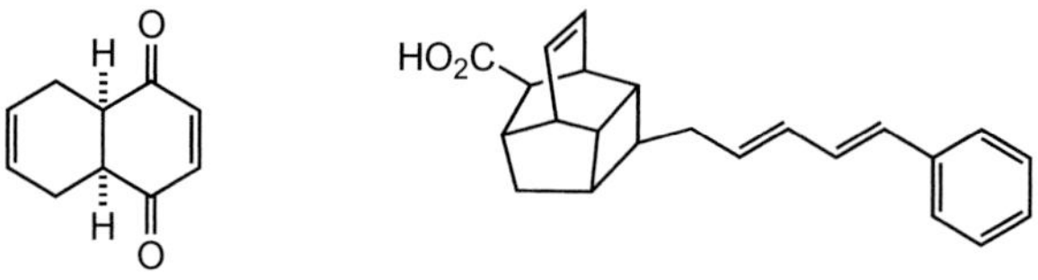

3. Pyrethrin I is a natural insecticide found in the seedcases of chrysanthe-mums and is used to make "mosquito coils." Label the stereocenters as "R" or "S" according to the Cahn-Ingold-Prelog system. Note the differences in the structure of this natural product and Nirmatrelvir. Devise a semi-synthesis of the bicyclic amino acid component of Nirmatrelvir starting from this abundant natural product.

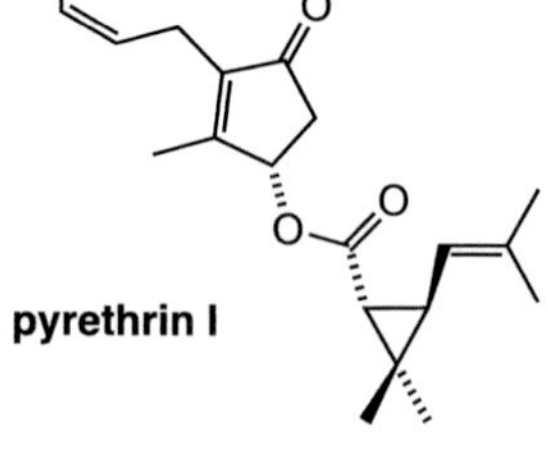

pyrethrin I

4. There are three cyclopropane disconnections that one could make on the natural product sesquicarene leading to reactive free carbene or carbenoid precursors. Critically analyze each path and decide which is the most promising. Explain your rationale. Propose a racemic synthesis of this natural product.

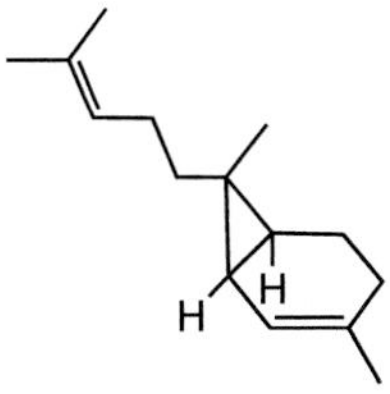

sesquicarene

5. Draw up a plan to synthesize racemic β-chamigrene from 2,6-heptanedione. Include a retrosynthetic analysis, labeling the retrons. Propose a synthetic route based on your analysis. (Hint: you will need to modify one of the functional groups β-chamigrene in order to reveal the key retron.)

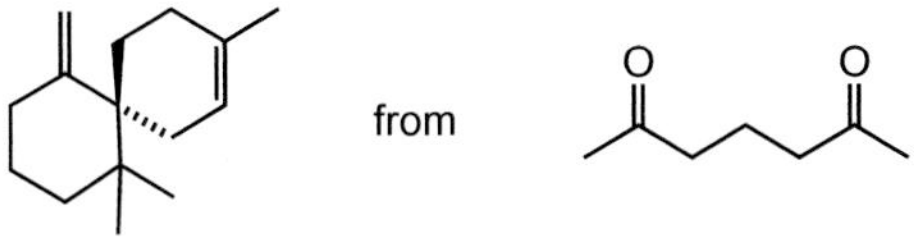

β-chamigrene   from

6. Which bond in the following compound would be the best to break following Corey's topological strategy for retrosynthetic disconnection? What functionality would you add the resulting structure to form the bond in the synthetic direction?

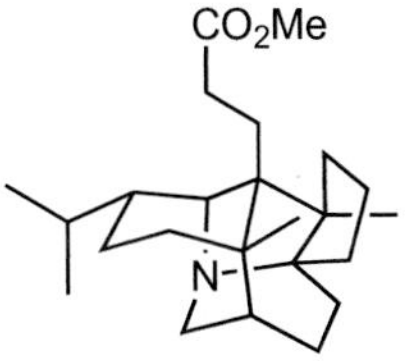

CO_2Me

7. Centrolobine is a tetrahydropyran-containing natural product that has been synthesized by several research groups. Using a chemically oriented database (such as SciFinder or Reaxys) or even a more general internet search engine (such as Google Scholar), find an example of its total synthesis that features a Prins cyclization. Next, find a synthesis that features another key

reaction. Which type of strategy categories do your found syntheses belong to (transform, structural, topological, stereochemical)?

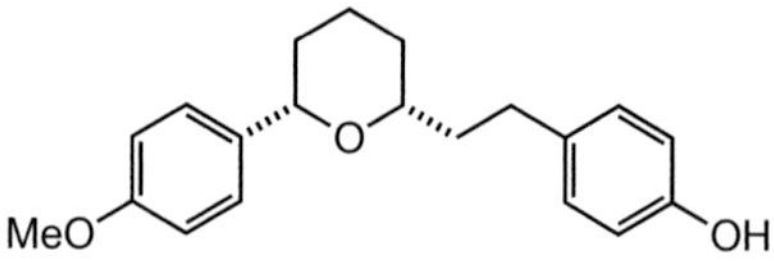

centrolobine

2 Vying for Control
The Synthesis of Reserpine and Quinine

CONCEPTS AND REACTIONS INTRODUCED IN CHAPTER 2:

- **The Bischler–Napieralski reaction** (Fodor, G., & Nagubandi, S. (1980). Correlation of the von Braun, Ritter, Bischler–Napieralski, Beckmann and Schmidt reactions via nitrilium salt intermediates. *Tetrahedron, 36*(10), 1279–1300.)
- **The Pictet–Spengler reaction** (Cox, E. D., & Cook, J. M. (1995). The Pictet–Spengler condensation: a new direction for an old reaction. *Chemical Reviews, 95*(6), 1797–1842.)
- **The Henry reaction** (Palomo, C., Oiarbide, M., & Laso, A. (2007). Recent advances in the catalytic asymmetric nitroaldol (Henry) reaction. *European Journal of Organic Chemistry, 2007*(16), 2561–2574.)
- **Meerwein–Pondorf–Verley reduction** (Nishide, K., & Node, M. (2002). Recent development of asymmetric syntheses based on the Meerwein–Pondorf–Verley reduction. *Chirality, 14*(10), 759767.)
- **Lemieux–Johnson oxidative cleavage** (Rajagopalan, A., Lara, M., & Kroutil, W. (2013). Oxidative alkene cleavage by chemical and enzymatic methods. *Advanced Synthesis & Catalysis, 355*(17), 3321–3335.)
- **Asymmetric catalytic Diels–Alder reactions** (Corey, E. J. (2002). Catalytic enantioselective Diels–Alder reactions: methods, mechanistic fundamentals, pathways, and applications. *Angewandte Chemie International Edition, 41*(10), 1650–1667.)
- **The Mitsunobu reaction** (T. Y. S., & Toy, P. H. (2007). The Mitsunobu reaction: origin, mechanism, improvements, and applications. *Chemistry–An Asian Journal, 2*(11), 1340–1355.)
- **The Swern oxidation** (Marx, M., & Tidwell, T. T. (1984). Reactivity-selectivity in the Swern oxidation of alcohols using dimethyl sulfoxide-oxalyl chloride. *The Journal of Organic Chemistry, 49*(5), 788–793.)
- **The Staudinger reaction** (Gololobov, Y. G., Zhmurova, I. N., & Kasukhin, L. F. (1981). Sixty years of Staudinger reaction. *Tetrahedron, 37*(3), 437–472.)
- **Asymmetric catalytic Michael reaction** (Hui, C., Pu, F., & Xu, J. (2017). Metal-catalyzed asymmetric Michael addition in natural product synthesis. *Chemistry–A European Journal, 23*(17), 4023–4036.)

DOI: 10.1201/9781003369431-2

- **Oxidation of alcohols using tetra-*n*-propylammonium perruthenate** (Griffith, W.P., Ley, S. V. (1990). TPAP: Tetra-*n*-propylammonium per-ruthenate, a mild and convenient oxidant for alcohols. *Aldrichimica Acta 23*(1), 13–19.
- **The Suzuki cross-coupling reaction** (Farhang, M., Akbarzadeh, A. R., Rabbani, M., & Ghadiri, A. M. (2022). A retrospective-prospective review of Suzuki–Miyaura reaction: From cross-coupling reaction to pharmaceutical industry applications. *Polyhedron 227*, 1–23.

RESERPINE

No study of organic synthesis would be complete without mentioning the contributions of R. B. Woodward, a prodigy of chemistry who achieved what might be considered "rock-star status" for his highly publicized natural product total syntheses and rather unorthodox lifestyle. His lectures were legendary, often spanning hours and consisting of a well-organized "chalk talk" (pre-PowerPoint) fueled by daiquiris and cigarettes. We will begin our discussion of the work of master synthetic chemists with Woodward's synthesis of the natural product reserpine.

Reserpine (Figure 2.1) is an alkaloid (an organic compound containing one or more amines) that is isolated from the Indian snakeroot (*Rauwolfia serpentina).* Snakeroot (*chandrika* in Sanskrit) has been used in traditional Indian medicine to treat a variety of conditions. About 50 bioactive substances have been isolated from this plant, of which reserpine is the most important. Although its value as a sedative has largely been superseded by other drugs, reserpine is still used to treat high blood pressure. From the synthetic standpoint, the molecule's fused ring system and six stereocenters presented quite a challenge. When Woodward published a full account of the total synthesis of reserpine in 1958,[1] it was considered a major accomplishment that demonstrated the power of organic synthesis at that time.

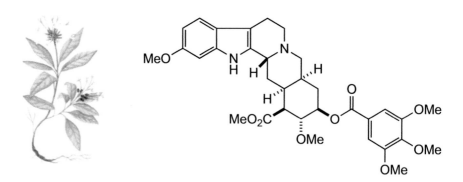

FIGURE 2.1.   *Rauwolfia serpentina* (left) and the structure of reserpine (right).

WOODWARD'S SYNTHESIS

Woodward's plan for the synthesis of reserpine was based on a combination of what we would call transform- and structure-based strategies (Figure 2.2). Labile bonds were identified and then broken in accordance with a particular transform in mind. These bond disconnections were performed in the order shown below in retrosynthetic fashion. The first disconnection involves an ester C–O bond and releases Compound **I**. This is followed by an iminium ion reduction that sets up the key Bischler–Napieralski transform. Note that the secondary alcohol in Ring E needs to be protected to assure chemoselectivity. Finally, a lactam bond is broken to give a secondary amine that can be made from Compounds **II** and **III** by reductive amination. Thus, Woodward reduced the reserpine synthesis problem to one of preparing three key building blocks—**I**, **II**, and **III**—then linking them together using known reactions. The Bischler–Napieralski reaction was used to form reserpine's C-ring. You may not be familiar with the Bischler–Napieralski reaction (a named reaction);

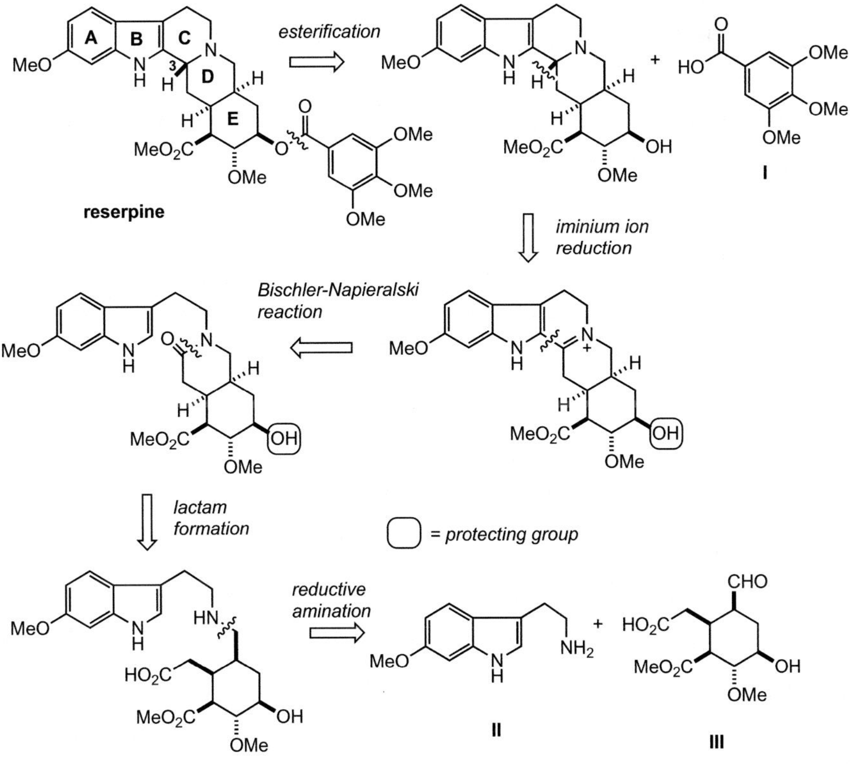

FIGURE 2.2. Woodward's plan for the synthesis of reserpine presented in retrosynthetic format.

its abridged mechanism is shown below in a "soft box." The substitution of indoles is an example of heteroelectrophilic electrophilc heteroaromatic.

> **Some advice:** Whenever you come across a reaction that you are unfamiliar with, it is a good idea to look it up (in a reference book, Google Scholar, or SciFinder) and write out a working mechanism for it. By "working mechanism," I mean one that enables you to understand what bonds are made/broken, what the reaction stoichiometry is, and whether the reaction will have any selectivity issues.

Just how one would control the stereochemistry at C3 of reserpine was not dealt with at this stage. As was often the case with Woodward's total syntheses, teams of coworkers pursued the target via multiple complimentary paths. The most efficient path to reserpine (in terms of step count) is presented here.

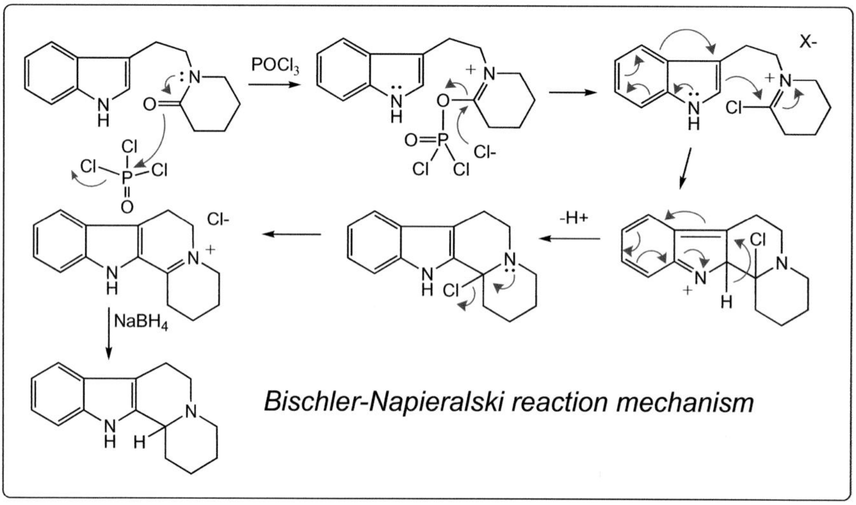

Bischler-Napieralski reaction mechanism

The synthesis begins with the preparation of 6-methoxytryptamine (Building Block **II**, Figure 2.3). A diazonium salt was formed from a readily available aniline, and this is reacted with formaldehyde oxime in the presence of copper (II) sulfate to give a substituted benzaldehyde after hydrolysis. This reaction proceeds through an aryl radical intermediate. This compound was then condensed with nitromethane to give a nitroalkene (the Henry reaction) that, upon hydrogenolysis, produced an aniline aldehyde that cyclizes to form the indole nucleus of reserpine. Aromatic acylation with oxalyl chloride introduces a two-carbon chain. After the reaction of

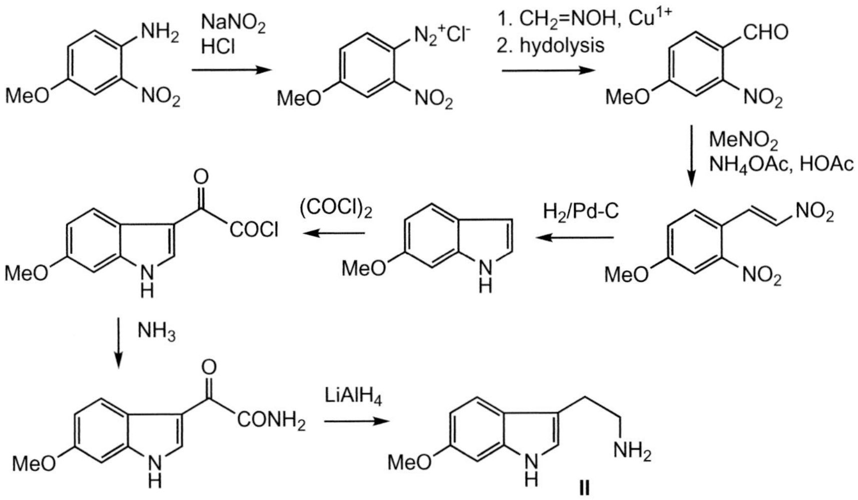

FIGURE 2.3. Woodward's synthesis of 6-methoxytryptamine (Building Block **II**).

the remaining acid chloride with ammonia, the primary and vinylogous amides are reduced with LiAlH$_4$ to give 6-methoxytryptamine (**II**).

The E-ring (Building Block **III**) presents a significant synthetic challenge because of its five contiguous stereocenters. Woodward took full advantage of both molecular orbital and conformational effects to control the configuration of the stereocenters in **III**. Synthesis of this building block (Figure 2.4) commenced with a Diels–Alder cycloaddition between benzoquinone and (E)-1-carbomethoxy-butadiene. At first glance, it might seem as though these two cycloaddition components (dienophile and diene, respectively) would seem to be poorly matched because they are both electron deficient. However, the benzoquinone is extremely electron deficient (its LUMO energy is estimated to be five eV lower than the LUMO of the reactive dienophile acrolein), so the reaction proceeds upon heating. As expected, this Diels–Alder reaction occurs via an *endo* transition state resulting in the correct stereochemistry for three of five cyclohexane substituents. Both ketones were then subjected to Meerwein–Pondorf–Verley reduction. This reaction has the Lewis acidic Al(i-PrO)$_3$ interacting with the ketone, thus setting up the intramolecular transfer of a hydride from an isopropoxy ligand to the substrate ketone. The process is reversible but can be driven forward by distilling off the acetone as it forms. When this reaction is forced to proceed in the reverse direction, the starting ketone becomes the substrate, and it is known as the Oppenhauer oxidation. Because the diketone has a cup-like shape, the hydride addition takes place on the less hindered convex face of the molecule. The three-dimensional (3-D) structure of the diketone, obtained from a molecular mechanics calculation with density functional theory refinement, is shown at the top of the figure with a 3-D rendering of the molecule to the right.

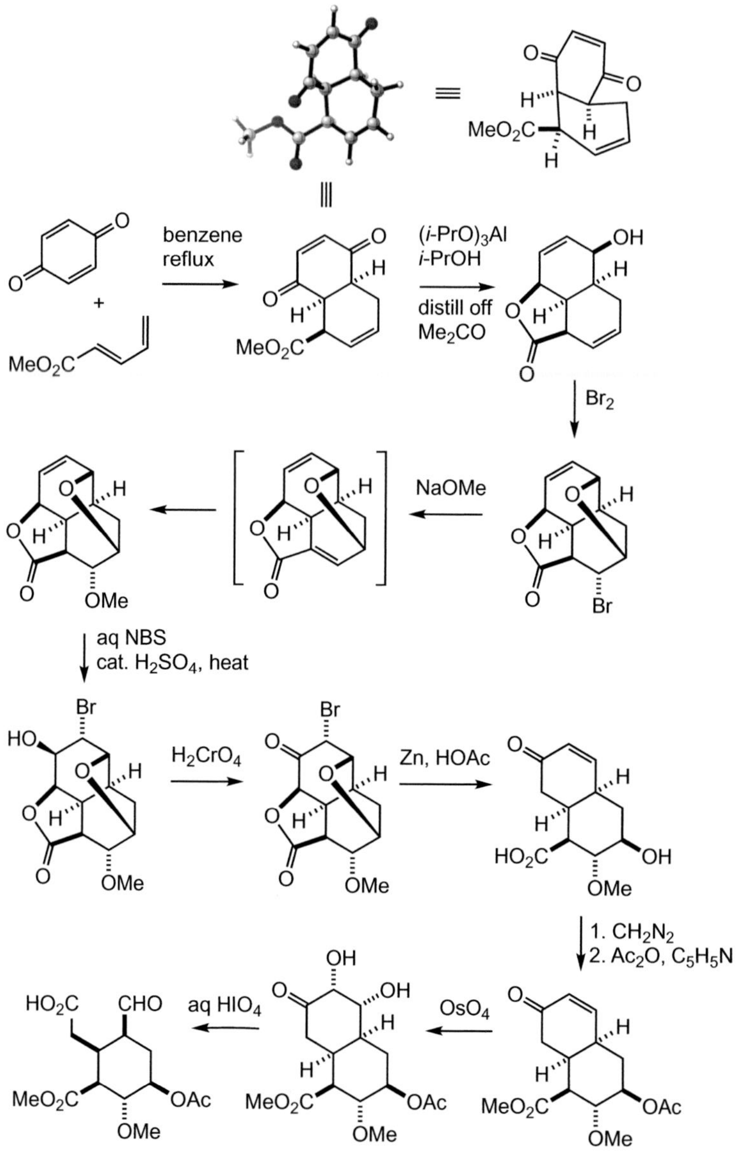

FIGURE 2.4. Woodward's synthesis of Building Block **III**.

More advice: During your study of organic synthesis, you will need to visualize 3-D renderings of molecules. You can do this with handheld molecular models or by using a molecular modeling program.

The alcohol that is proximal to the ester undergoes an intramolecular transesterification reaction to give a γ-lactone (via an entropically favored five-membered ring transition state) that serves to protect both the alcohol and carboxylic acid. Treatment with bromine selectively forms an intermediate bromonium ion (via its reaction with the more electron-rich alkene) that is intercepted by the free alcohol (favoring an axial approach) to give a bromoether. Exposure of this compound to sodium methoxide leads to β-elimination of HBr to give the α,β-unsaturated lactone that then undergoes the conjugate addition of methanol, also on the convex face, to install the methoxy group stereoselectively.

Meerwein-Pondorf-Verley reduction mechanism

Attention then turned to the manipulation of the remaining alkene. Bromination under harsher aqueous reaction conditions resulted in the regioselective and stereoselective formation of a bromohydrin. The selectivity of this reaction can be attributed to the axial attack of the intermediate bromonium ion by water. This reaction serves to protect the alcohol that would eventually be connected to Building Block **I**. Jones oxidation of the free alcohol produced a ketone that had bromide and carboxylate leaving groups at the α- and α'-positions, setting the stage for two reductive elimination reactions that are initiated by metallic zinc in acetic acid. These reactions proceeded through zinc enolates and resulted in the formation of a cyclohexenone. The carboxylic acid was converted to a methyl ester with diazomethane, and the alcohol was acetylated with acetic anhydride. Cis-dihydroxylation of the enone with osmium tetraoxide followed by periodic acid induced cleavage (the Lemieux–Johnson reaction) with loss of CO_2 formed the carboxymethyl and formyl E-ring substituents. It is constructive to consider the most stable conformation of this molecule; note that four of the five contiguous substituents on the cyclohexane chair occupy equatorial positions.

The stage was now set to assemble the pentacyclic core of reserpine (Figure 2.5). The sequence began with a reductive amination of the indole amine (AB-ring system) and the cyclohexyl aldehyde (Ring E), followed by lactam formation to install Ring D. Exposure to phosphorous oxychloride initiated the Bischler–Napieralski sequence, producing the pentacyclic iminium ion. However, iminium reduction with sodium borohydride did not produce the expected reserpine core but, rather, the "iso"-reserpine system with a 3S configuration instead of the natural 3R configuration. Clearly, hydride addition appeared to be under stereoelectronic control with axial attack being favored. Note that in iso-reserpine, the indole substituent on the piperidine ring is in the more stable equatorial configuration.

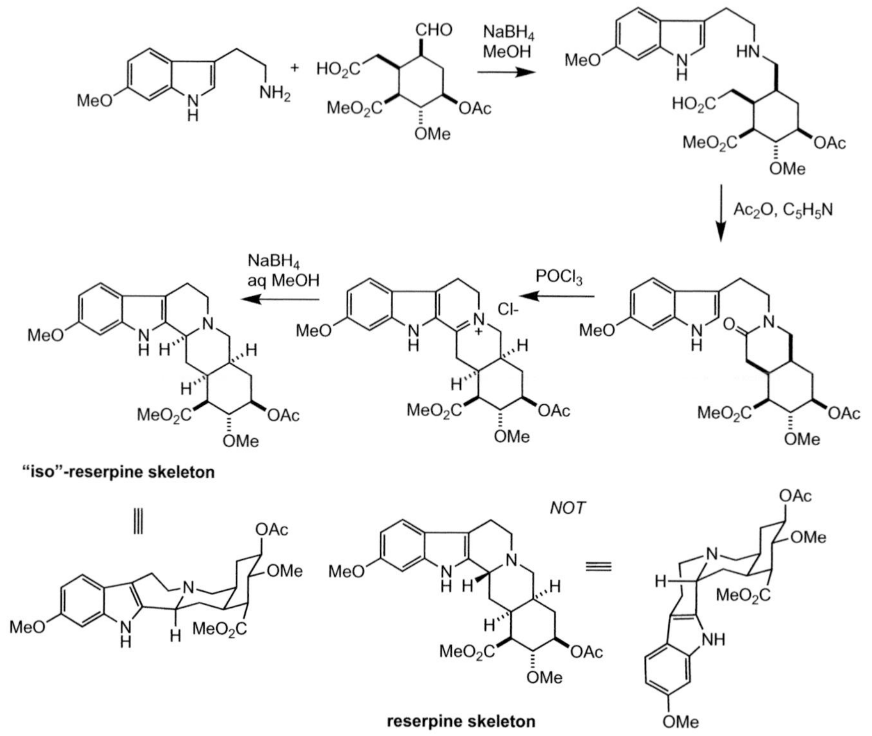

FIGURE 2.5.   Woodward's initial attempt to synthesize the reserpine core.

Woodward solved this problem by forcing the cis-fused D and E chairs in the pseudo-cis-decalin system to "flip" conformations (interchanging the axial and equatorial positions), producing a molecule that forced the bulky indole ring to occupy an axial position (Figure 2.6). This transformation was accomplished by saponifying the ester functional groups to unveil a γ-hydroxy acid that could be cyclized to a γ-lactone with the dehydrating reagent dicyclohexyl carbodiimide. Acid-catalyzed epimerization corrected the C3 stereocenter, and methanolysis restored the E-ring methyl ester and hydroxyl group. Based on the elegant mechanistic work of Joule, which demonstrated that 3-deuterio-isoreserpine undergoes acid-catalyzed epimerization without loss of label,[2] this epimerization probably occurs via breaking and reforming of the transannular bond as shown for reserpine itself. The effect that the lactone bridge has on the piperidine ring conformation may be visualized by comparing truncated handheld models of the hydroxyl acid and the lactone. With the C3

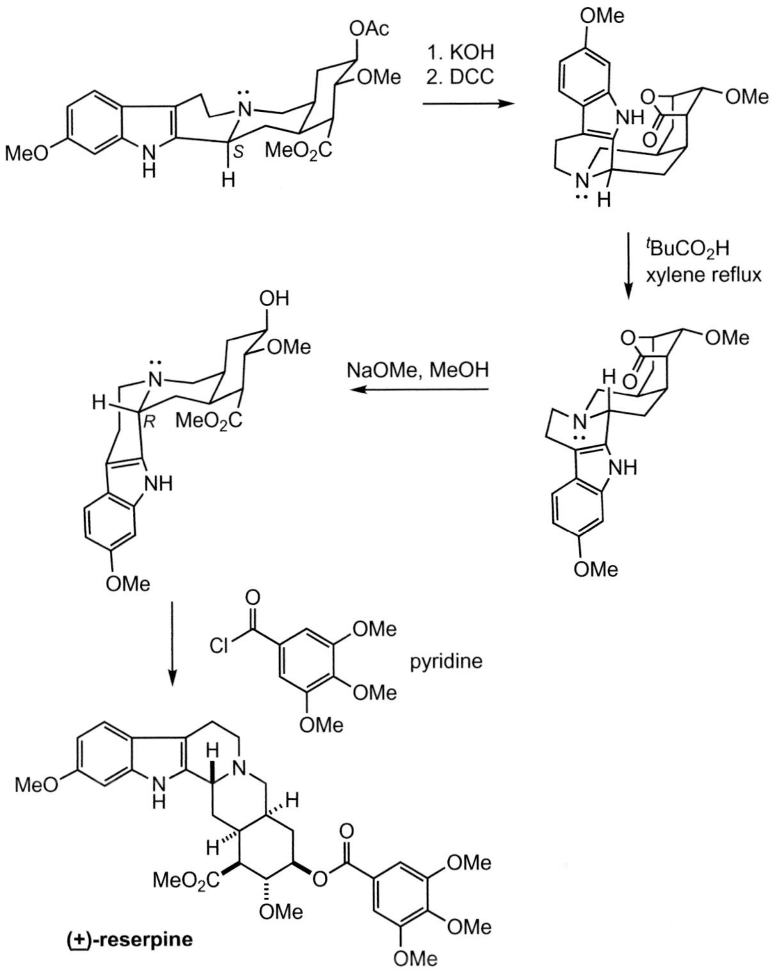

FIGURE 2.6. The final stages of Woodward's synthesis of racemic reserpine.

configuration secure, the final Building Block (**I**) was attached to the free alcohol by acylation with trimethylgalloyl chloride to give racemic reserpine, which was separated into its antipodes by classical resolution using camphorsulfonic acid as the resolving agent. Preparation of the levorotatory before antipode, whose physical data matched that of the natural substance, concluded Woodward's total synthesis of reserpine.

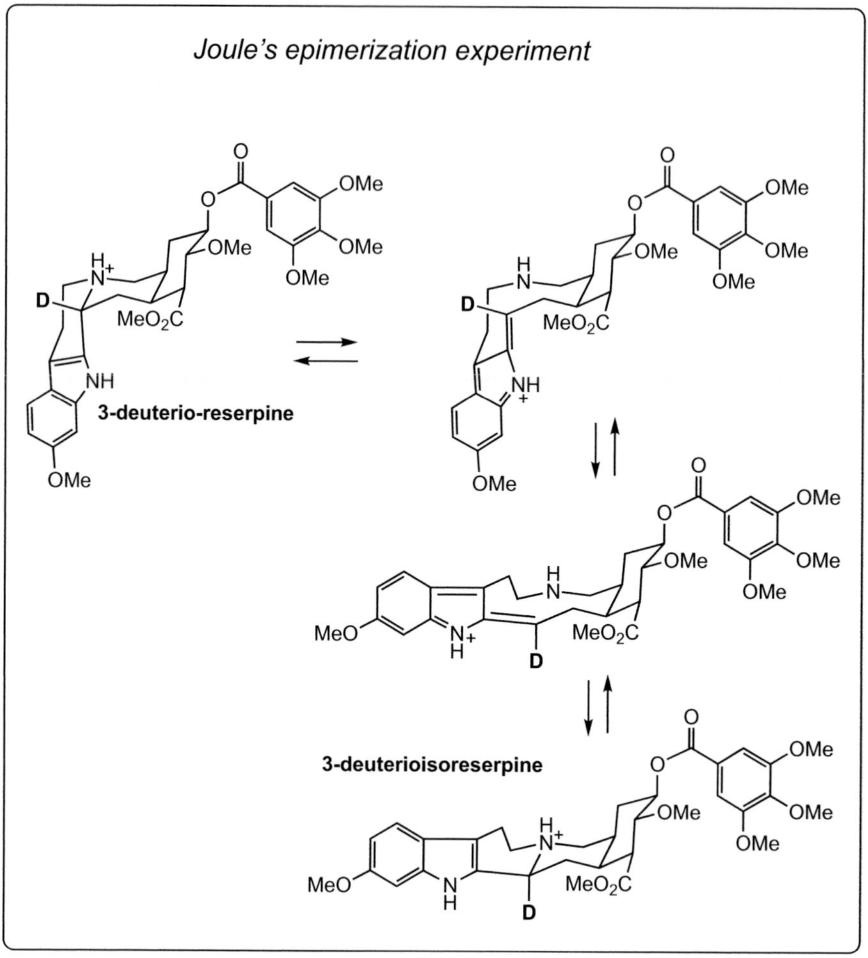

Joule's epimerization experiment

3-deuterio-reserpine

3-deuterioisoreserpine

JACOBSEN'S APPROACH

In the interim, since Woodward's 1958 report, many labs have tried to improve and modernize the synthesis of reserpine. Notable efforts include Gilbert Stork's use of a stereoelectronically controlled Pictet–Spengler reaction to set the stereochemistry at C3 as opposed to Woodward's use of a conformational lock to enforce thermodynamic stereocontrol. A conceptually simple solution to the C3 stereochemistry problem would employ the indole as the nucleophile in an irreversible Pictet–Spengler reaction. This was Stork's approach,[3] will be covered in the tutorial at the end of this chapter. In 2013, Eric Jacobsen reported an enantioselective synthesis of the unnatural antipode of reserpine.[4] The synthesis showcased the use of asymmetric organocatalysis to set the developing stereochemistry, including the recalcitrant C3 stereocenter. The key organocatalyzed formal aza Diels–Alder reaction (that is, a

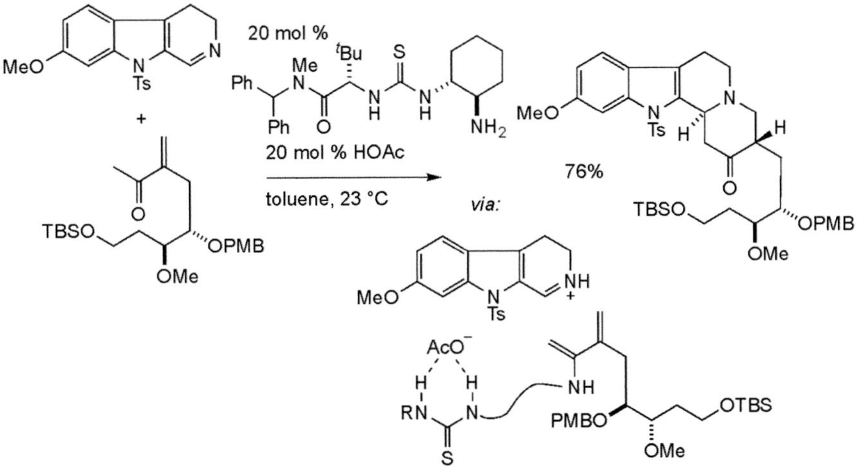

FIGURE 2.7. The key organocatalyzed aza Diels–Alder reaction in Jacobsen's synthesis of ent-reserpine.

Diels–Alder reaction in which the diene or dienophile has nitrogen substituents) that produced the correct relative C3 stereochemistry is shown in Figure 2.7.

In terms of efficiency, Woodward's synthesis of racemic reserpine was accomplished in 20 steps from benzoquinone. With eight construction steps, plus a bonus step for the Diels–Alder reaction, its ideality (Id) was 45%. Of course, half of the material that was made, as well as the reagents, solvents, etc., was wasted on the unwanted enantiomer. Jacobsen's synthesis of the unnatural enantiomer of reserpine circumvented this problem by employing an enantioselective reaction to make the starting material, was accomplished in 20 steps, and had an Id of 50%. Thus, although the methodology and approach to stereocontrol differed, the overall efficiency was roughly equivalent by this measure. As we shall see at the end of this chapter, Stork's more or less classical approach to reserpine clearly outperforms these earlier syntheses.

QUININE

Quinine is a naturally occurring alkaloid found in the bark of the *Cinchona pubescens*, a tree found in the montane forests of Bolivia, Colombia, Costa Rica, Ecuador, Panama, Peru, and Venezuela (Figure 2.8). It was introduced to Europe by Spanish Jesuits as a treatment for malaria, giving Spain a monopoly on the natural product. After obtaining cinchona seeds surreptitiously, the Dutch colonial government set up plantations in Indonesia and controlled the world's supply of quinine at the start of the Second World War. The supply line to allied countries was cut when Indonesia came under Japanese control. An alternative source of this drug was urgently needed, as allied military operations were being conducted in areas where malaria was endemic.

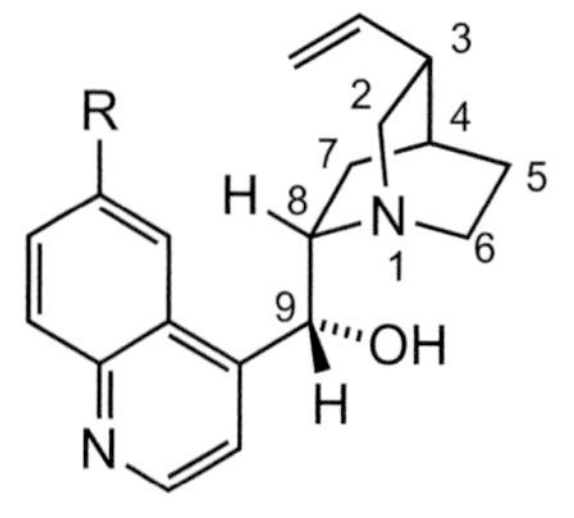

quinine (R = OMe)
cinchonidine (R = H)

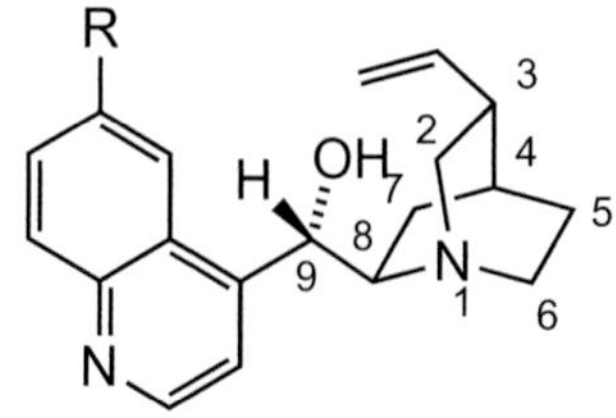

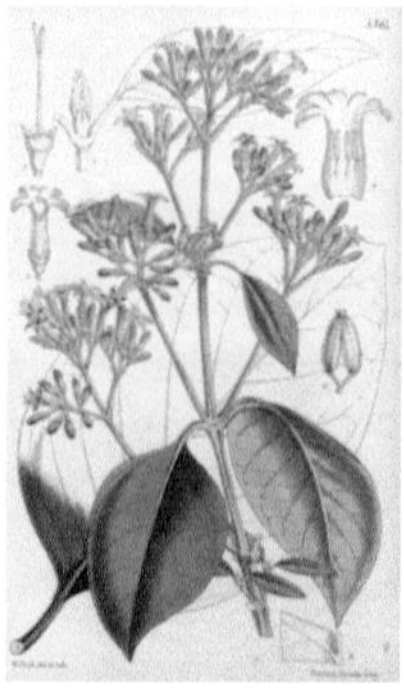

quinidine (R = OMe)
cinchonine (R = H)

FIGURE 2.8.   Botanical illustration of *Cinchona pubescens* and the chemical structures of quinine and related alkaloids.

STORK'S SYNTHESIS

Chemists had been investigating the structure and reactions of quinine since the mid-1800s. Pasteur had converted quinine to quinotoxine and Rabe had converted quinotoxine back to a mixture of quinine and three other stereoisomers (Figure 2.9). However, it was well into the next century before quinine was synthesized in the lab. Woodward and William von Eggers Doering reported the synthesis of quinotoxine in 1944, which constituted a formal synthesis of quinine, as Rabe had reported the conversion of the former to the latter. Their achievement received considerable publicity, but it did not solve the supply problem. In fact, doubt as to whether Rabe (and by association Woodward) ever prepared quinine from quinotoxine was only cleared up in 2001 when Robert Williams (a former student of Woodward) repeated Rabe's experiment and proved, using modern analytical methods, that Rabe had indeed succeeded in making quinine. We shall discuss two more recent syntheses of quinine, starting with Gilbert Stork's work[5] and begin our analysis by noting the problems associated with Rabe's approach. Like Woodward, Stork was also a master at recognizing key disconnections and synthetic planning by taking into account the 3-D structural features of the target molecule.

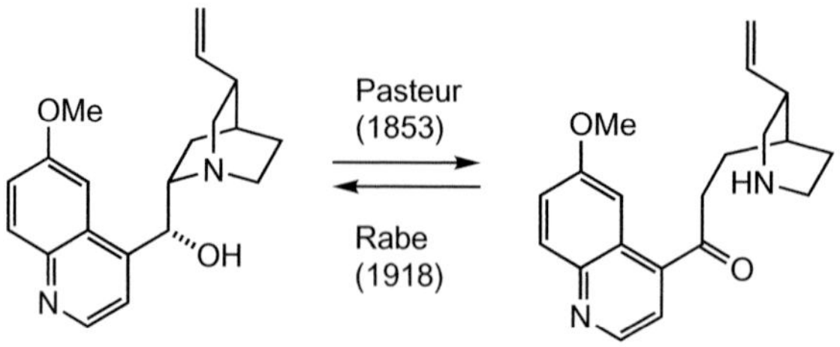

Pasteur
(1853)

Rabe
(1918)

FIGURE 2.9.   Known chemical conversions of quinine and quinotoxine.

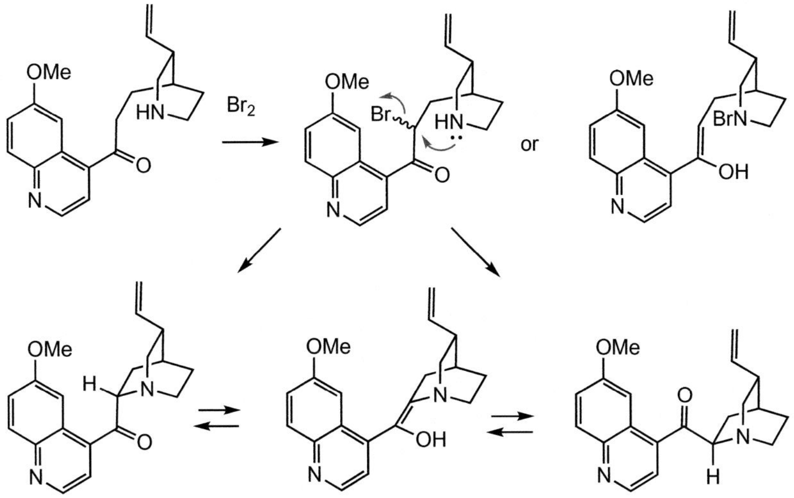

FIGURE 2.10. Rabe's mutarotation problem.

One of the problems associated with reliance on Rabe's reported conversion of quinotoxine to quinine was the propensity of the α-aminoketone intermediate, prepared by bromination of quinotoxine followed by the S_N2 displacement of the bromide, to undergo epimerization via the enol (Figure 2.10). This was the source of two of the three undesired stereoisomers that were produced in his synthesis along with quinine during the nonselective reduction of the ketone.

As seen from a retrosynthetic perspective (Figure 2.11), Stork circumvented this problem by avoiding the troublesome ketone altogether and making what, at first, seems to be a rather unorthodox quinuclidine N1–C6 bond disconnection. This bond cleavage violates the topological strategy rule (described in Chapter 1) that prioritizes bond breaking to eliminate stereocenters. The more logical disconnection was to break the N1–C8 bond as per Rabe and then Woodward. Stork's genius was that he homed in on the key problem that plagued prior synthetic efforts and perceived that breaking the N1–C6 bond would produce a piperidine ring with equatorial substituents at C2, C4, and C5 (piperidine numbering). His recognition of this hidden structural pattern enabled him to set the C2 stereocenter by stereoelectronically controlled axial addition of hydride to an iminium ion. Coupled with the stereoselective benzylic hydroxylation developed by Milan Uskokovic's group at Hoffmann-La Roche, he would be able to access quinine without going through the configurationally labile α-aminoketone intermediate.

The key iminium ion was to be derived from an azidoketone that would be formed by oxidation of an azido alcohol, the configuration of which was inconsequential. This secondary alcohol was to be obtained by the nucleophilic addition of an organolithium species to an aldehyde that contained all atoms and two of the stereocenters that make up quinine's quinuclidine ring.

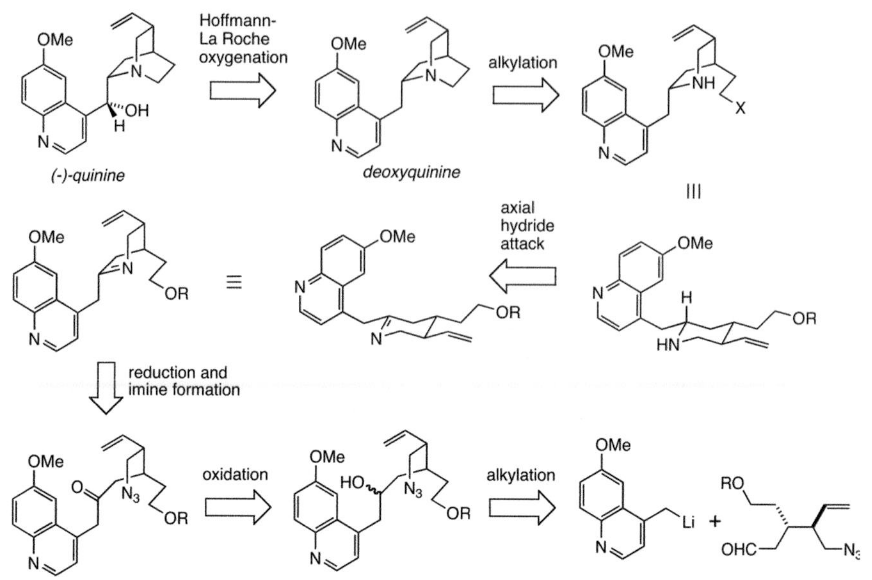

FIGURE 2.11. Stork's retrosynthetic analysis of quinine.

The preparation of this azidoaldehyde (Figure 2.12) deserves comment. It is available in eight steps from the readily available (S)-Taniguchi lactone.[6] Lewis acid-catalyzed ring opening with diethylamine gave an acyclic amidoalcohol that was protected as a *t*-butyl dimethylsilyl (TBS) ether. The lithium enolate of this compound was alkylated with the *t*-butyldiphenylsilyl (TBDPS) ether of 2-iodoethanol to give the 2,3-disubstituted amide. It should be noted that direct alkylation of the Taniguchi lactone was deemed less satisfactory than the longer sequence that proceeded through the diethylamide.

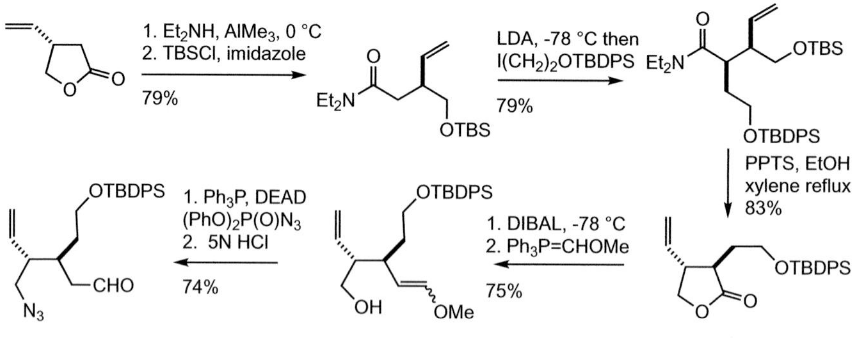

FIGURE 2.12. Synthesis of the azidoaldehyde from the (S)-Taniguchi lactone.

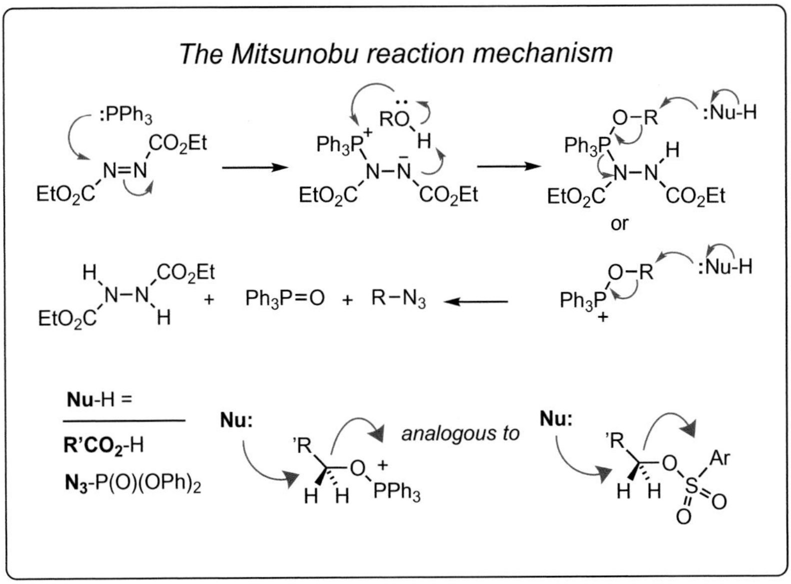

The Mitsunobu reaction mechanism

:PPh₃
CO₂Et
N=N
EtO₂C

→

RO
Ph₃P⁺ H
N–N
EtO₂C CO₂Et

→

O–R :Nu-H
Ph₃P
N–N H
EtO₂C CO₂Et

or

H CO₂Et
N–N + Ph₃P=O + R–N₃ ←
EtO₂C H

O–R :Nu-H
Ph₃P
+

Nu-H =

R'CO₂-H

N₃-P(O)(OPh)₂

Nu:
'R
O +
H H PPh₃

analogous to

Nu:
'R
O Ar
H H S=O
O

Acid-catalyzed relactonization, which involved selective removal of the TBS group in the presence of the more stable TBDPS ether, was followed by semi-reduction to the lactol with diisobutylaluminum hydride (DIBAL). This lactol was in equilibrium with the tautomeric hydroxy aldehyde, which could be trapped by a methoxymethylene phosphonium ylide to give a mixture of enol ethers. This variation on the Wittig reaction has general utility. It starts out with an aldehyde and ends up, after hydrolysis of the initially formed enol ether, with a new aldehyde that is one methylene unit longer. Finally, the free primary alcohol was converted to an azide (a masked amine) using Mitsunobu conditions, and the enol ether was hydrolyzed to the homologated aldehyde.

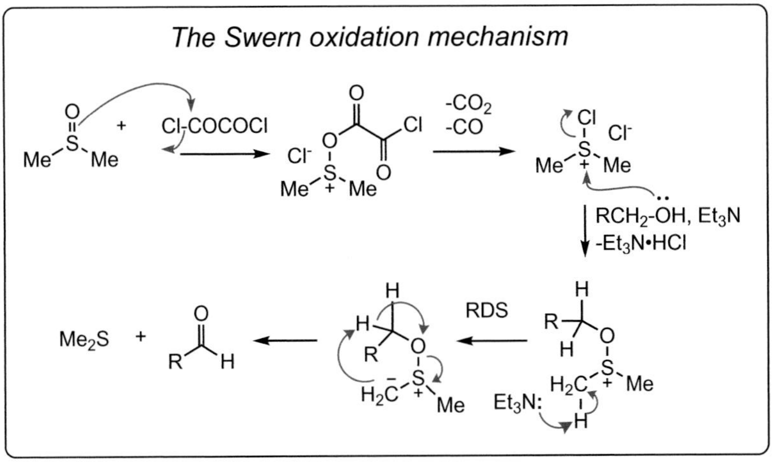

The Swern oxidation mechanism

O
S   + Cl-COCOCl
Me Me

→

Cl O
S
Me + Me O O Cl

-CO₂
-CO
→

Cl Cl⁻
S
Me + Me

| RCH₂-OH, Et₃N
↓ -Et₃N•HCl

Me₂S +
O
R H

←

H
H O
R S
H₂C + Me Et₃N:

RDS
←

H
R O
H
H₂C + S Me
H

Et₃N:
H

The next phase of the synthesis was concerned with the convergent assembly of the quinine skeleton (Figure 2.13). Deprotonation of 6-methoxy-4-methylquinoline with lithium diisopropylamide (LDA) at the acidic benzylic position produced a lithiated species that added to the azido aldehyde to give a mixture of secondary alcohols that were oxidized to a common ketone by Swern oxidation. The azide was reduced with triphenylphosphine via a Staudinger reaction, which produced an imine. Sodium borohydride reduction of this imine delivered hydride axially to give the desired (2S, 4S, 5R) configured trisubstituted piperidine. Note that all three piperidine substituents are in the energetically favored equatorial position, a consequence of making the initial N1–C6 disconnection. The stage was now set to complete the synthesis of quinine.

The synthetic finale (Figure 2.14) began with conversion of the protected alcohol to a primary mesylate that, upon heating, underwent an S_N2 reaction to give deoxyquinine. Application of the Hoffmann-La Roche hydroxylation conditions, which involved the reaction of a benzylic anion or radical with oxygen, produced quinine in 16 linear steps from the Tamiguchi lactone. Stork's stereocontrolled synthesis of quinine solved a long-standing problem that the previous syntheses simply ignored. His prescient recognition that the stereochemical problems associated with Rabe's approach could be avoided by making an apparently counterintuitive bond disconnection was the key to success.

JACOBSEN'S SYNTHESIS

In 2004, Jacobsen reported an asymmetric catalytic synthesis of quinine.[7] This synthesis illustrates the impact that methodological advances can have on synthetic strategy. Thus, he rescued Rabe's original N1–C8 disconnection, leading to a very effective synthesis of the target molecule. His retrosynthetic analysis (Figure 2.15) features the ring opening of an (8S, 9S) epoxide by a 3,4-disubstituted piperidine to simultaneously generate the quinuclidine ring system and install the C9 alcohol stereospecifically. The epoxide was derived from a vicinal diol prepared using a Sharpless asymmetric dihydroxylation reaction. The quinoline moiety would be attached to a disubstituted piperidine by a palladium catalyzed Suzuki

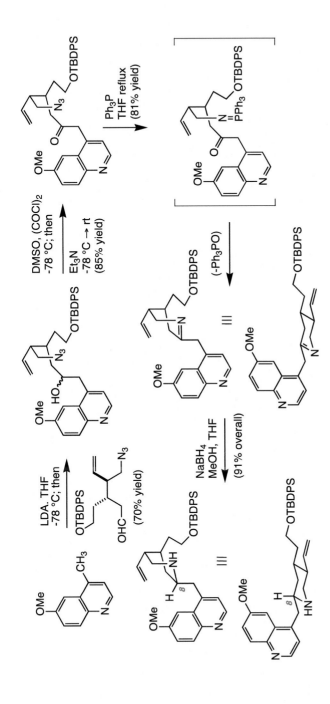

FIGURE 2.13.   Stork's assembly of the quinine skeleton.

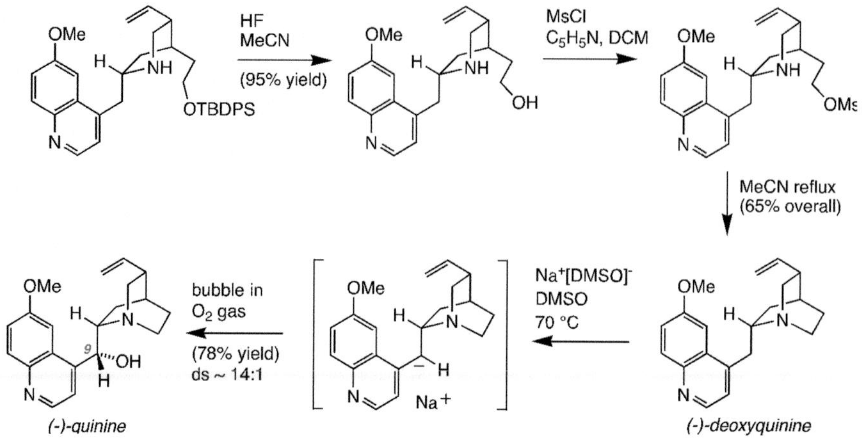

FIGURE 2.14.   Stork's quinine end game.

cross-coupling reaction, and the piperidine would arise from an asymmetric cata-lytic Michael addition.

In the forward direction (Figure 2.16), the synthesis starts out with a Horner–Wadsworth–Emmons reaction to give an α, β-unsaturated imide. This substrate underwent an enantioselective Michael addition of methyl cyanoacetate that is cata-lyzed by a chiral Al(III)-salen complex. However, the reaction produced a mixture of nitrile diastereomers favoring the wrong stereoisomer. These nitrile diastereomers were not separated but reduced to their corresponding amines wherein they cyclized to give a mixture of δ-lactams, favoring the undesired β-diastereomer. The ratio of

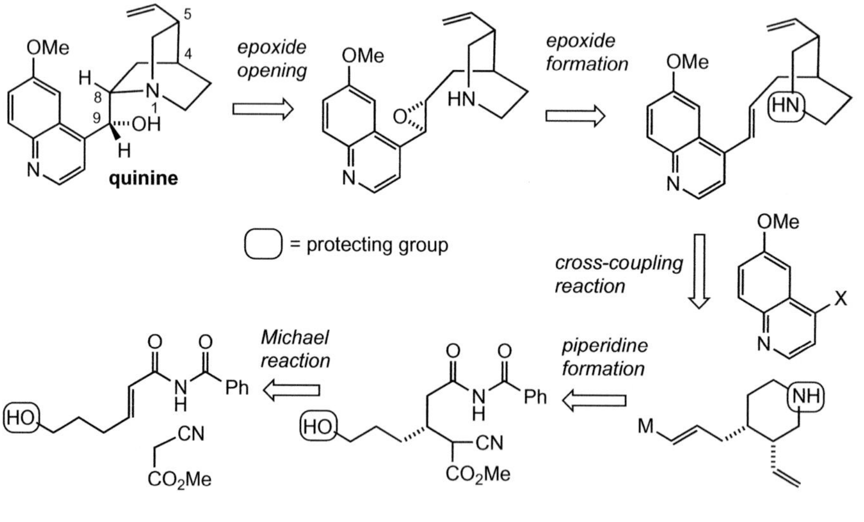

FIGURE 2.15.   Retrosynthetic analysis of Jacobsen's quinine synthesis.

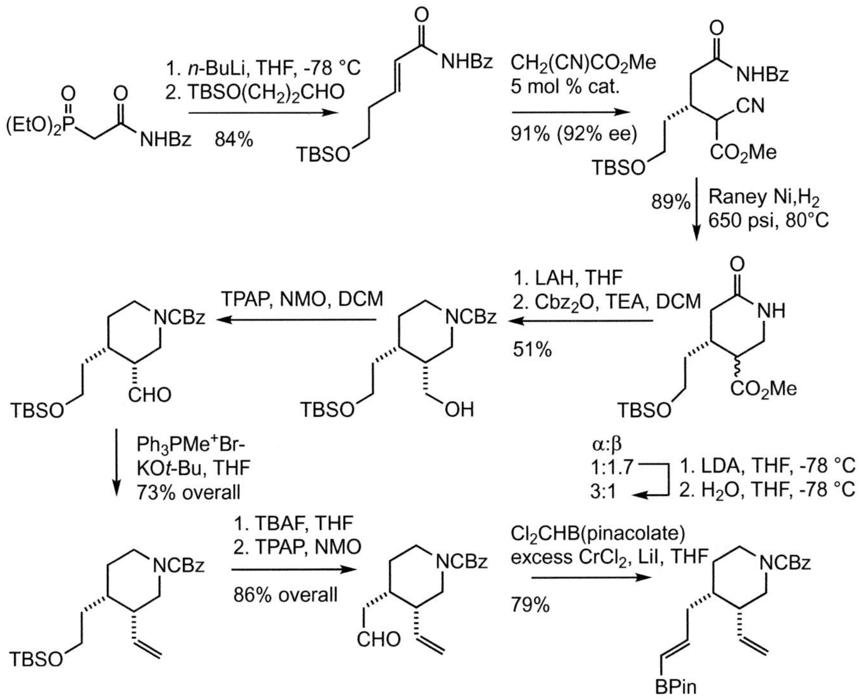

FIGURE 2.16. Jacobsen's synthesis of the 3,4-disubstituted piperidine ring.

diastereomeric lactams could be reversed by kinetic protonation of the derived lithium ester enolate. Lithium aluminum hydride reduced both the ester and the lactam to give a mixture of aminoalcohols that was N-protected with a benzyloxycarbonyl (Cbz) group. Controlled oxidation of the major alcohol using Ley's tetrapropylammonium perruthenate (TPAP) reagent produced an aldehyde that was converted to a vinyl group via a Wittig reaction with $Ph_3P = CH_2$. The perruthenate reagent is the mildest oxidizing agent in the series $Os(VIII) > Ru(VIII) > Cr(VI) > Ru(VII)$. Its utility is the selective oxidation of primary alcohols to aldehydes without going further to the carboxylic acid level and not reacting with secondary alcohols. The TBS ether was removed with tetrabutylammonium fluoride, and the resulting primary alcohol was oxidized to an aldehyde that was converted to an (E)-vinyl boronate with a Takai reagent. The stage was set for Suzuki cross-coupling to an isoquinoline derivative.

Jacobsen's quinine endgame is shown in Figure 2.17. The starting 4-bromo-6-methoxyquinoline was prepared by bromination of the known 6-methoxyquinolinone. The final sequence began with the palladium-catalyzed Suzuki cross-coupling of this bromide and the vinylic boronate, which produced the quinoline-conjugated (E)-alkene. This Pd(0)-catalyzed cross-coupling reaction, along with the related Stille and Negishi couplings to be covered in the next chapter, have proven to be

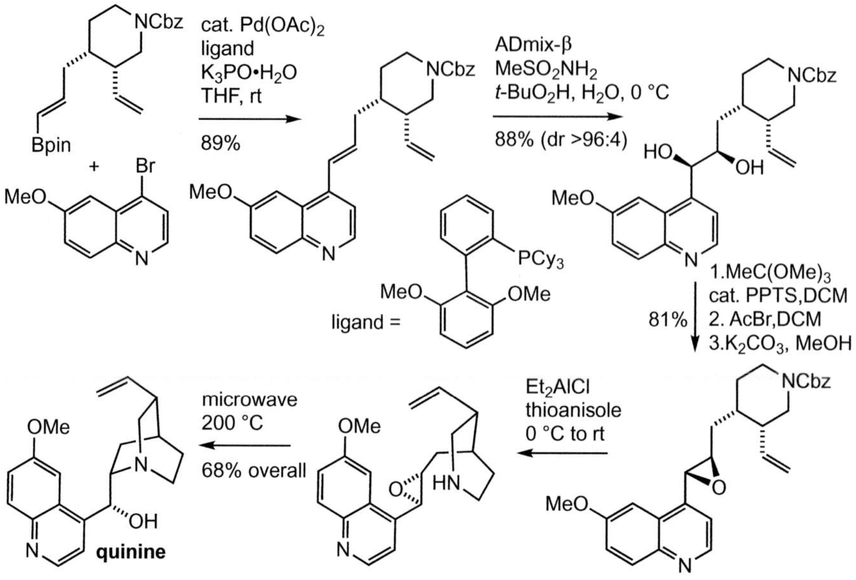

FIGURE 2.17.   Jacobsen's endgame in his enantioselective synthesis of quinine.

very useful for organic synthesis. All three of these reactions can be understood as variations on the common mechanistic theme, which is shown below, wherein R^1–X may be considered the electrophilic partner and R^2–M the nucleophilic partner. In this way, the transition metal Pd enables the direct displacement of C(sp2)–X bonds, which is not possible using standard nucleophiles. Asymmetric epoxidation of this alkene failed to give satisfactory results, so an indirect route to this key intermediate was taken. Thus, chemoselective Sharpless asymmetric dihydroxylation using the dihydroquinoline-derived ADmix-β reagent produced the (8R, 9R)-diol in good yield and high diastereoselectivity and did not react with the terminal olefin.[8] This diol was converted to the corresponding epoxide using the one-pot procedure developed by Sharpless.[9] The Cbz protecting group was removed with a strong Lewis acid (hydrogenolysis would also reduce the vinyl group) and microwave-induced opening of the epoxide afforded quinine in 16 steps from the starting β-silyloxypropionaldehyde. By substituting the quinine-derived ADmix-α for ADmix-β, the diastereomeric natural product quinidine could be obtained by the same route.

General mechanistic scheme for palladium catalysed cross coupling reactions

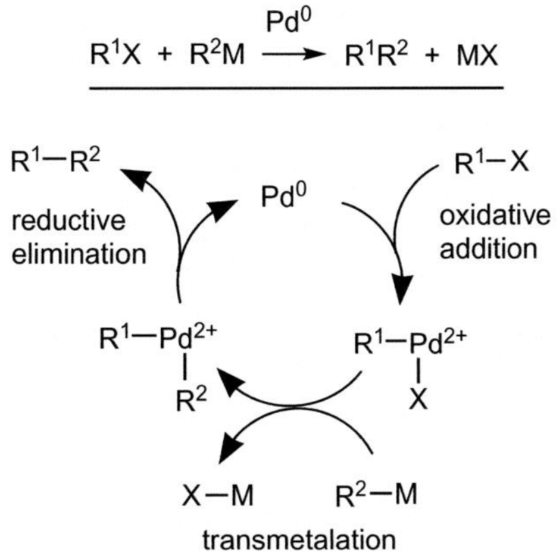

$$R^1X + R^2M \xrightarrow{Pd^0} R^1R^2 + MX$$

R^1-R^2
reductive elimination

Pd^0

R^1-X
oxidative addition

R^1-Pd^{2+} | R^2

R^1-Pd^{2+} | X

$X-M$ R^2-M
transmetalation

Empirical model for the Sharpless asymmetric dihydroxylation

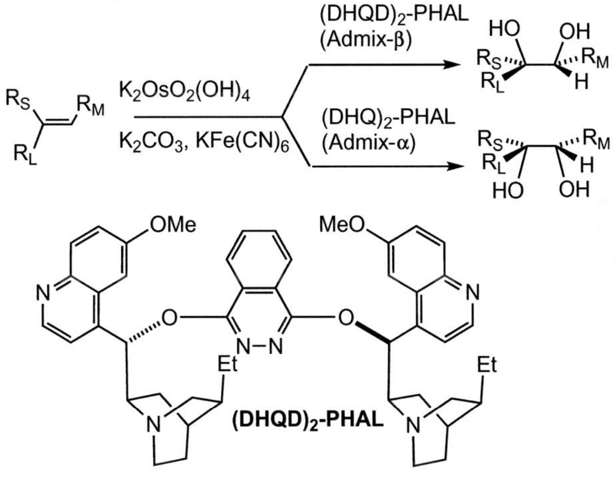

(DHQD)$_2$-PHAL
(Admix-β)

$K_2OsO_2(OH)_4$

K_2CO_3, KFe(CN)$_6$

(DHQ)$_2$-PHAL
(Admix-α)

(DHQD)$_2$-PHAL

Stereoretentive conversion of vicinal diols to epoxides

Regarding efficiency, the Stork and Jacobsen syntheses of quinine were roughly equivalent (16 and 15 steps, ideality = 50% and 47%, respectively) using our revised ideality formula. However, their approaches differed in terms of both the strategy and tactics that were employed, reflecting methodological advances that had been made in the area of asymmetric catalysis.

TUTORIAL: THE PICTET–SPENGLER (P–S) REACTION AND RETRON PATTERN RECOGNITION

Six reactions that involve the addition of a nucleophile (Nu:) to an iminium ion (RHC =N$^+$R'R") are shown in Figure 2.18, differing only in the type of nucleophile that is involved. Their corresponding retrons are shown in magenta. You probably were introduced to the reductive amination and Strecker synthesis in your undergraduate organic chemistry course. The Mannich reaction, which involves an enol nucleophile, was introduced in Chapter 1 in the context of Robert Robinson's tropinone synthesis. Phenols, which have an enol substructure of sorts, can also act as nucleophiles as in the Betti reaction. If one tethers the phenol component to the amine component as shown, the product is a tetrahydroisoquinoline. This substructure is found in numerous alkaloid natural products and pharmaceuticals. Likewise, indoles can be tethered to an amine, and the resulting condensation with aldehydes produces the β-carboline skeleton. These two reactions may be thought of as the prototypical Pictet–Spengler reactions.

RESERPINE REVISITED

Reserpine contains a β-carboline substructure, thus begging the question of whether the Pictet–Spengler reaction could be used for the synthesis of this natural product. In the Woodward synthesis of reserpine, we saw that a hydride nucleophile prefers to attack the Bischler–Napieralski iminium from its axial α-face due to stereoelectronic effects resulting in the isoreserpine structure (Figure 2.6). In a beautiful piece of work that illustrates the logic of a master's synthetic plan combined with the travails

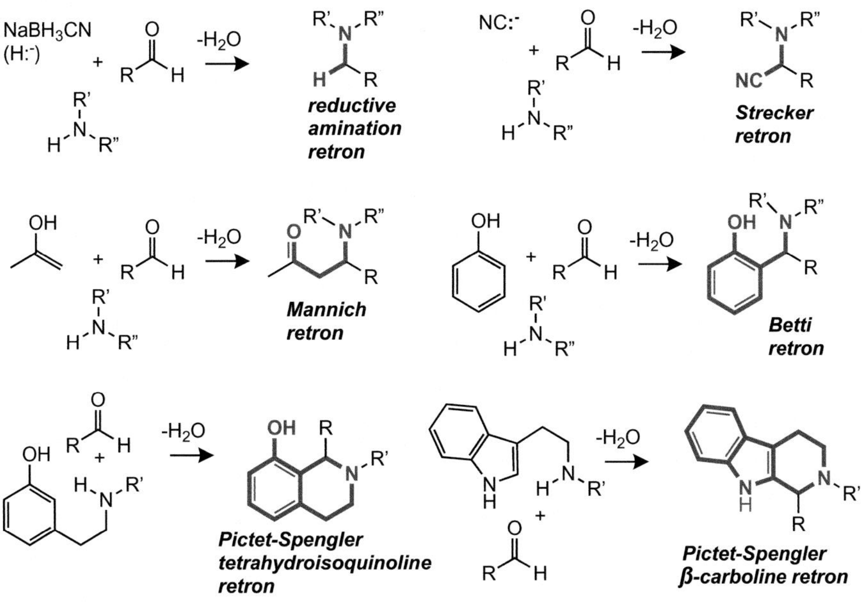

FIGURE 2.18. Reactions and retrons associated with imines and iminium ions.

associated with its execution, we now describe Gilbert Stork's synthesis of reserpine. Stork realized that the Pictet–Spengler nucleophile (C2 of the indole) would also prefer an axial approach to the cyclic iminium and that this would result in the natural reserpine structure (Figure 2.19). The tetracyclic iminium would be formed by the condensation of 6-methoxytryptamine with an aldehyde tosylate. The aldehyde functional group could be masked by engaging with the C1 alcohol via a lactone linkage which is the retron for a Baeyer–Villiger reaction. Application of this transform led to a bicyclo[2.2.2]octane system that could arise from a formal (4 + 2) cycloaddition process such as a Diels–Alder reaction (R = Me$_3$Si) or a double Michael reaction (R = M), though the latter reaction might be more likely to succeed, as the Diels–Alder components do not seem to be particularly activated. Besides being a retron for the Baeyer–Villiger reaction, the lactone serves as a protecting group for the C1 alcohol, thus enabling selective O-methylation of the C2 alcohol.

The actual synthesis (Figure 2.20) began with a double Michael reaction between the kinetic enolate of 4-benzyloxymethylcyclohexenone and the pictured β–silyl acrylate. Deprotonation under nonequilibrating conditions (LDA at low temperature in tetrahydrofuran (THF)) produced the less substituted kinetic enolate which added to the β-carbon of the acrylate, resulting in an ester enolate that underwent an intramolecular Michael addition to the newly formed enone. The choice of a silane-based alcohol surrogate that could be converted to the target's methoxy group was a response to the facile β-elimination of methoxide that was observed when β-methoxyacrylate was used as the Michael acceptor. Like the analogous oxidation of an alkyl borane to an alcohol, the conversion of a silane to an alcohol proceeds through

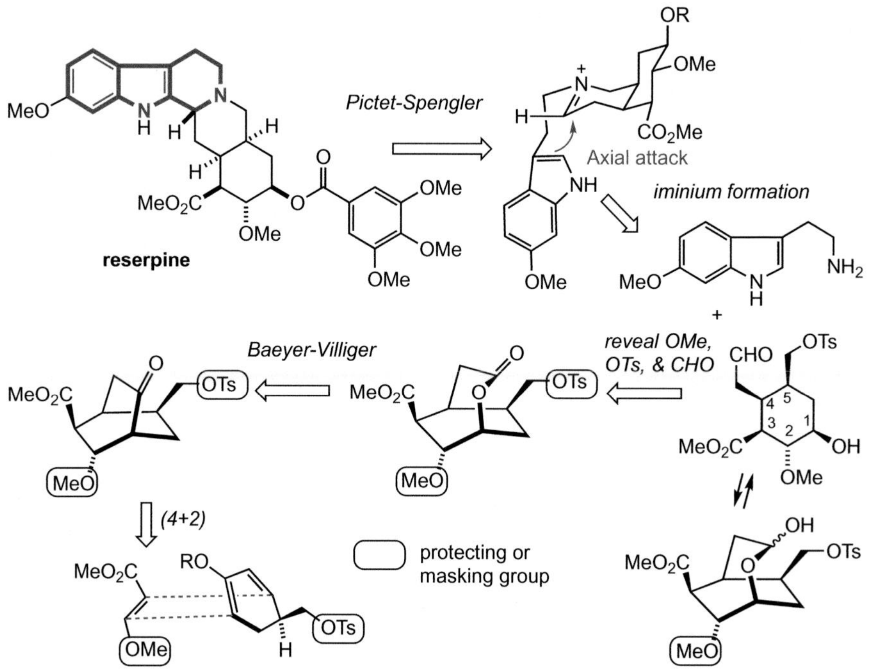

FIGURE 2.19. Stork's plan for the synthesis of reserpine.

a hypervalent species akin to a tetrahedral intermediate resulting from nucleophilic addition to a ketone or aldehyde. Thus, in one key step, the bicyclo[2.2.2]octan-2-one was produced in high yield as a single stereoisomer. The observed stereochemistry is consistent with the beznzyloxymethyl substituent blocking one face of the dienolate in the first Michael addition and bridging of the lithium enolate and enone carbonyl controlling the stereochemistry in the second Michael reaction. The overall reaction may also be viewed as an enolate-accelerated, endo-selective Diels–Alder reaction.

The next three steps effected functional group interchanges. First, the furanyl group was replaced by a fluorine atom, producing a more reactive fluorosilane. Then, the benzyl ether was replaced with a tosylate. The resulting ketone was treated with buffered meta-chloroperbenzoic acid (MCPBA) to give the bridging lactone. The lactone was partially reduced to its lactol, which opened spontaneously to the aldehyde tosylate, the substrate for the key Pictet–Spengler reaction. When this compound was treated with an excess of potassium cyanide (KCN) followed by 6-methoxytryptamine, a single aminonitrile was obtained in high yield. Exposure of this compound to hydrochloric acid (HCl) resulted in formation of the desired iminium ion and Pictet–Spengler reaction producing a pentacycle with the correct C3 stereochemistry. Finally, esterification with 3,4,5-trimethoxybenzoyl chloride gave racemic reserpine. The synthesis was repeated using enantiomerically pure 4-benzyloxymethylcyclohexenone to give (-)-reserpine.

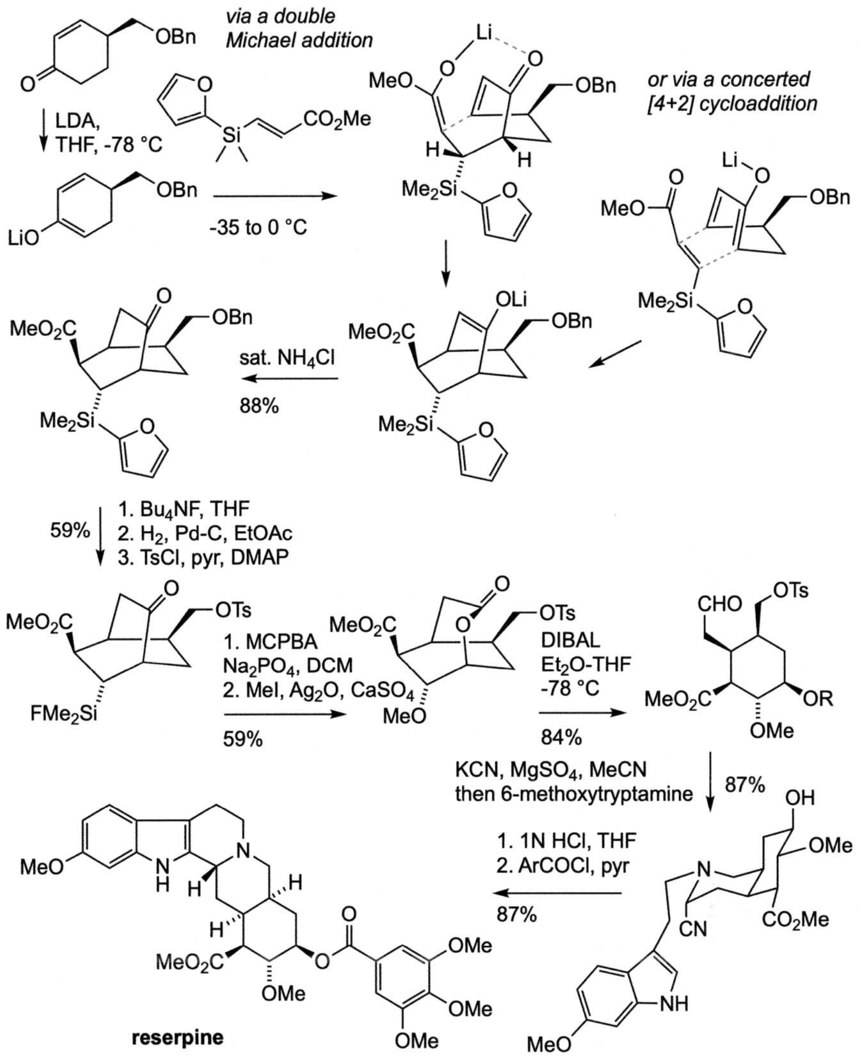

FIGURE 2.20. Gilbert Stork's synthesis of reserpine.

The Stork synthesis of reserpine proceeded in ten steps from 4- benzyloxymethyl-cyclohexenone with an overall yield of 19%. The ideality of this synthesis was 70%, making it the most efficient of the three reserpine syntheses covered in this chapter, providing that one starts counting steps with the enone. Nine additional steps were required to make this substrate from commercially available pantolactone, so the actual efficiency is much lower.

As is often the case with total syntheses, the original plan ran into trouble when an attempt was made to put it into practice. The full story is instructive. Thus, when

6-methoxytryptamine was first combined with the aldehyde tosylate, a pentacycle was generated but as a mixture of C3 epimers favoring the undesired epimer (Figure 2.21). It was reasoned that this outcome resulted from the preferential attack of the indole ring on an initially formed disubstituted imine, a Pictet–Spengler reaction that did not benefit from the stereoelectronic control of a cyclic iminium ion. Furthermore, the pentacyclic C3 epimers were known to equilibrate to a mixture that favored the isoreserpine structure via transannular bond cleavage/reformation (see Woodward's synthesis). This posed a serious problem for the project, as the main objective was stereocontrol at this position. The reaction was then performed in the presence of excess cyanide to trap the disubstituted imine as an aminonitrile (a Strecker reaction) that would displace the tosylate before it reacted with the indole. However, when this

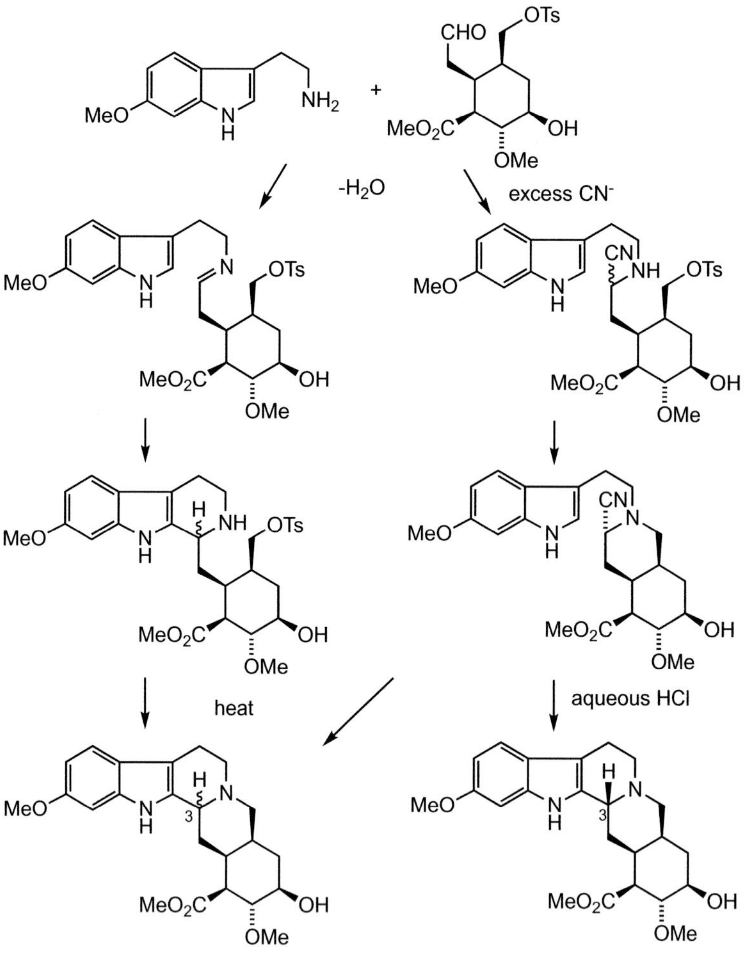

FIGURE 2.21. Unexpected problems and a mechanistically guided solution.

compound was heated, the isoreserpine stereochemistry still predominated. Further reasoning suggested that the aminonitrile had, indeed, produced the expected cyclic iminium salt but that the cyanide counterion formed a tight ion pair that blocked the α-approach of the indole nucleophile. In support of this hypothesis, simply exposing the aminonitrile to aqueous HCl—conditions that do not favor ion pairing—opened the α-face of the iminium for axial attack by the indole and produced the natural reserpine structure. This example shows how a reasonable synthetic plan can be successfully implemented using mechanistically guided rationales to circumvent unexpected problems.

ECTEINASCIDIN 743

Finally, a striking example that illustrates how multiple variations of the Pictet–Spengler reaction can be used to build tetrahydroisoquinolines (THIQs) comes from Corey's synthesis of the anticancer natural product Ecteinascidin (ET) 743 (Figure 2.22).[10] The first of three THIQs was assembled from a substituted phenylalanine that contained all three Pictet–Spengler reaction components: an electron-rich aromatic, an aldehyde, and a urethane-protected amine. Note that the aromatic substitution regioselectivity need not be ortho to a phenolic hydroxyl group. In the presence of a strong Lewis acid, a very reactive N-acyliminium species is generated and trapped by the electron-rich aromatic ring, producing an appropriately functionalized AB-ring THIQ. This is followed by a second Pictet–Spengler reaction that employs trifluoromethanesulfonic acid to generate the N-acyliminum intermediate that goes on to give the CDE-ring system. Finally, the FG-ring THIQ is formed diastereoselectively by the silica gel catalyzed P–S condensation of a substituted 2-phenylethylamine with a reactive α-ketoester.

SUMMARY

This chapter discussed classic syntheses of reserpine and quinine by R. B. Woodward and Gilbert Stork, as well as more recent syntheses of these natural products by Eric Jacobsen. The chapter's tutorial featured the Pictet–Spengler reaction, a time-honored method for the synthesis of β-carbolines as well as tetrahydroisoquinolines and showed its application to the synthesis of the reserpine as well as the structurally complex alkaloid ET-743. Woodward's synthesis of reserpine employed relatively simple reagents in reactions that could be readily scaled up. A drawback of the work was the fact that the synthesis necessarily produced racemic material, requiring a classical resolution to obtain enantiomerically pure reserpine. The highlight of this classic work was Woodward's ingenious manipulation of molecular conformation to control the critical C3 stereocenter of the natural product. Stork cleverly took advantage of the stereoelectronically preferred axial attack of nucleophiles onto endocyclic iminium ions in his elegant syntheses of reserpine and quinine. In both cases, enantioselectivity was achieved by starting with a simple, readily available chiral starting material. Jacobsen promoted a different approach to these natural products that utilized asymmetric catalysis for the enantioselective syntheses of ent-reserpine

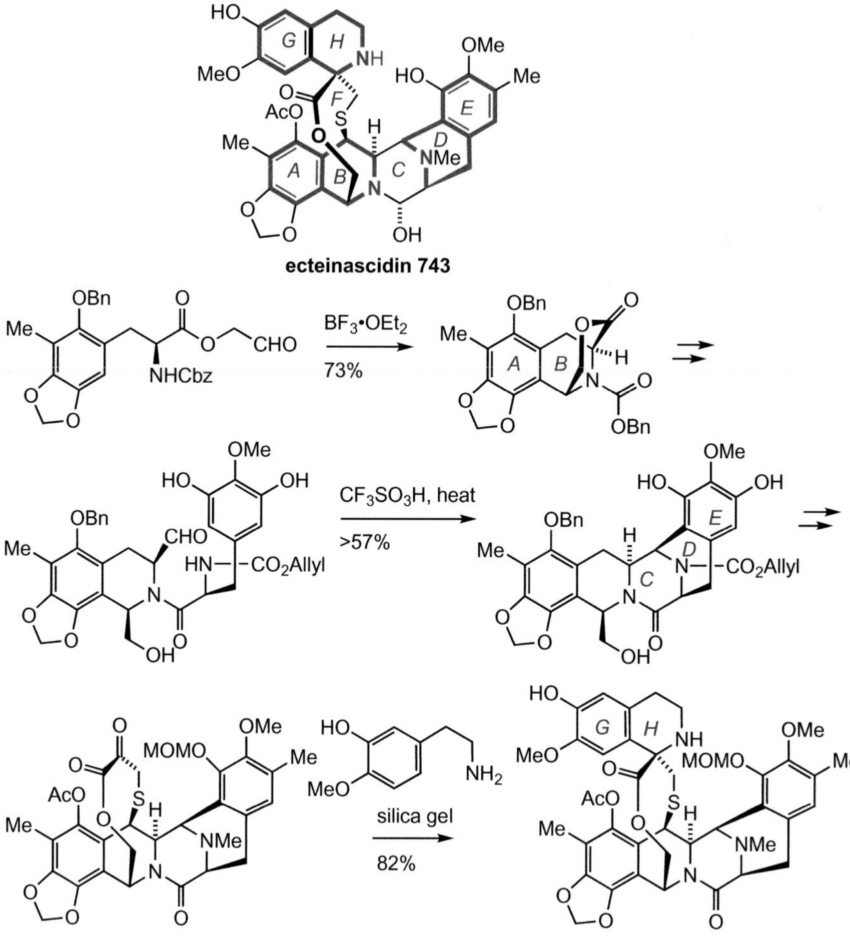

ecteinascidin 743

FIGURE 2.22. Three Pictet–Spengler reactions that were used to build tetrahydroisoquinolines in Corey's synthesis of ET-743.

and quinine. Both approaches have their merits. The classical approach may be more appropriate for synthesis of a specific target, whereas an approach based on asymmetric catalysis may be better suited for the construction of analog libraries with deep-seated structural variations as desired for diversity-oriented synthesis projects.

REFERENCES

1. Woodward, R. B., Bader, F. E., Bickel, H., Frey, A. J., & Kierstead, R. W. (1956). The total synthesis of reserpine. *Journal of the American Chemical Society*, 78(9), 2023–2025.
2. Gaskell, A. J., & Joule, J. A. (1967). The acid catalysed C3 epimerization of reserpine and deserpidine. *Tetrahedron*, 23(10), 4053–4063.

3. Stork, G., Tang, P. C., Casey, M., Goodman, B., & Toyota, M. (2005). Regiospecific and stereoselective syntheses of (±)-reserpine and (−)-reserpine. *Journal of the American Chemical Society*, *127*(46), 16255–16262.
4. Rajapaksa, N. S., McGowan, M. A., Rienzo, M., & Jacobsen, E. N. (2013). Enantioselective total synthesis of (+)-reserpine. *Organic Letters*, *15*(3), 706–709.
5. Stork, G., Niu, D., Fujimoto, A., Koft, E. R., Balkovec, J. M., Tata, J. R., & Dake, G. R. (2001). The first stereoselective total synthesis of quinine. *Journal of the American Chemical Society*, *123*(14), 3239–3242.
6. von Kieseritzky, F., Wang, Y., & Axelson, M. (2014). Facile production scale synthesis of (S)-Taniguchi lactone: A precious building-block. *Organic Process Research and Development*, *18*(5), 643–645.
7. Raheem, I. T., Goodman, S. N., & Jacobsen, E. N. (2004). Catalytic asymmetric total syntheses of quinine and quinidine. *Journal of the American Chemical Society*, *126*(3), 706–707.
8. Xu, D., Crispino, G. A., & Sharpless, K. B. (1992). Selective asymmetric dihydroxylation (AD) of dienes. *Journal of the American Chemical Society*, *114*(19), 7570–7571.
9. Kolb, H. C., & Sharpless, K. B. (1992). A simplified procedure for the stereospecific transformation of 1, 2-diols into epoxides. *Tetrahedron*, *48*(48), 10515–10530.
10. Corey, E. J., Gin, D. Y., & Kania, R. S. (1996). Enantioselective total synthesis of ecteinascidin 743. *Journal of the American Chemical Society*, *118*(38), 9202–9203.

PRACTICE PROBLEMS

1. Perform a retrosynthetic analysis of 4-amino-3-nitroanisole, the starting material for Woodward's reserpine synthesis. Identify retrons for each transform.

2. Write out a stepwise mechanism for each of the reactions in the following synthetic sequence.

3. The pyrrole ring of indole undergoes electrophilic heteroaromatic substitution at C3, whereas pyrrole itself undergoes substitution at C2. Using resonance structures, provide a rationale for this divergent behavior.

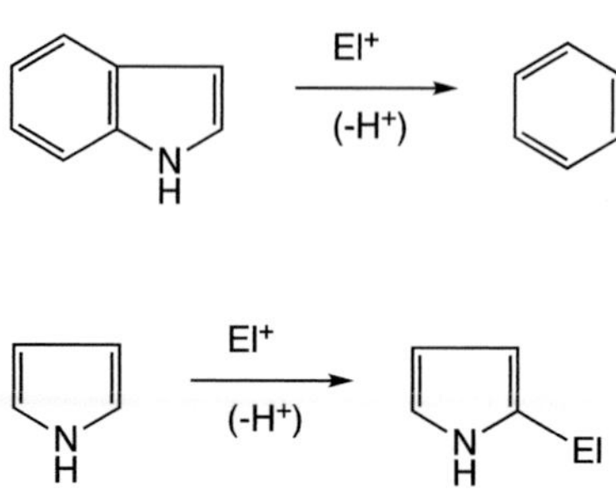

4. In the Bischler–Napieralski reaction that was used in Woodward's reserpine synthesis, why did the electrophilic carbon end up covalently bound to C2 of the indole?

a. Write out an arrow-pushing mechanism for the acid-catalyzed epimerization of the C3 stereocenter in Woodward's reserpine synthesis.

b. How could you modify a single reaction in Woodward's synthesis of racemic reserpine to make the synthesis enantioselective?

c. Propose a synthesis of the following molecule from readily available starting materials.

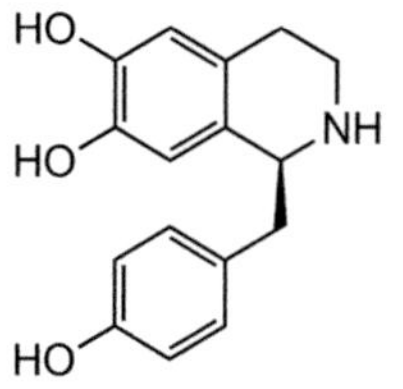

5. Propose a mechanism for the epimerization of isoreserpine and reserpine that is consistent with the following sets of experiments.

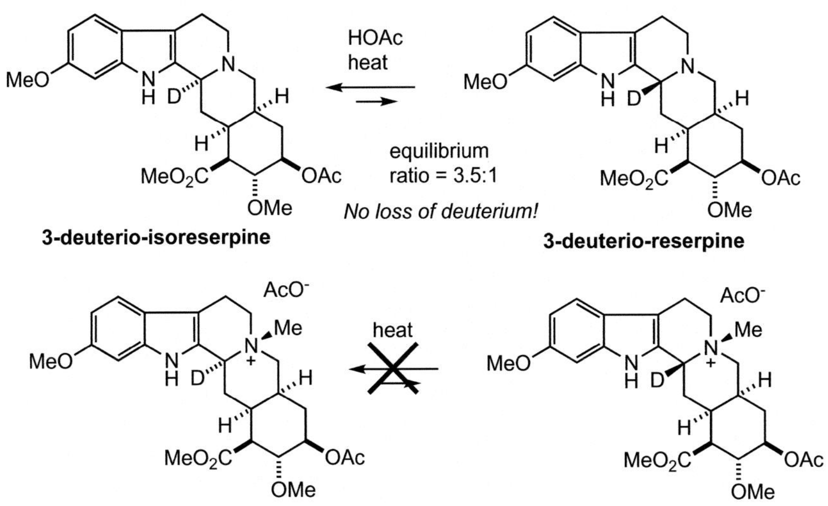
MeO
HOAc
heat
equilibrium
ratio = 3.5:1
No loss of deuterium!
MeO₂C
OAc
OMe
3-deuterio-isoreserpine
3-deuterio-reserpine
AcO⁻
Me
heat

3 A Helping Hand from Nature? Bioinspired Synthesis and Semi-synthesis

CONCEPTS AND REACTIONS INTRODUCED IN CHAPTER 3:

- **Biomimetic polyolefin cyclizations** (Yoder, R. A., & Johnston, J. N. (2005). A case study in biomimetic total synthesis: polyolefin carbocyclizations to terpenes and steroids. *Chemical Reviews*, *105*(12), 4730–4756.)
- **The modern interpretation of the Wittig reaction mechanism** (Byrne, P. A., & Gilheany, D. G. (2013). The modern interpretation of the Wittig reaction mechanism. *Chemical Society Reviews*, *42*(16), 6670–6696.)
- **Johnson variant of the Claisen rearrangement** (Fernandes, R. A., Chowdhury, A. K., & Kattanguru, P. (2014). The orthoester Johnson–Claisen rearrangement in the synthesis of bioactive molecules, natural products, and synthetic intermediates—recent advances. *European Journal of Organic Chemistry*, *2014*(14), 2833–2871.)
- **Barton–McCombie deoxygenation** (McCombie, S. W., Motherwell, W. B., & Tozer, M. J. (2004). The Barton–McCombie reaction. *Organic Reactions*, *77*, 161–432.)
- **The Hajos–Parrish–Eder–Sauer–Wiechert reaction** (List, B., & Turberg, M. (2019). The Hajos–Parrish–Eder–Sauer–Wiechert reaction. *Synfacts*, *15*(02), 0200. https://www.thieme-connect.com/products/ejournals/pdf/10.1055/s-0037-1612037.pdf)
- **Pericyclic reactions in organic synthesis** (Nicolaou, K. C., & Petasis, N. A. (1984). Pericyclic reactions in organic synthesis and biosynthesis: synthetic adventures with endiandric acids A–G. In *Strategies and Tactics in Organic Synthesis* (Vol. 1, pp. 155–173). Academic Press.)
- **Olefin metathesis reactions** (Hoveyda, A. H., & Zhugralin, A. R. (2007). The remarkable metal-catalysed olefin metathesis reaction. *Nature*, *450*(7167), 243–251.)
- **Metal-catalyzed cross coupling reactions.** Diederich, F., & Stang, P. J. (Eds.). (2008). *Metal-catalyzed cross-coupling reactions.* John Wiley & Sons.

   DOI: 10.1201/9781003369431-3

- **The Diels–Alder reaction in total synthesis** (Nicolaou, K. C., Snyder, S. A., Montagnon, T., & Vassilikogiannakis, G. (2002). The Diels–Alder reaction in total synthesis. *Angewandte Chemie International Edition, 41*(10), 1668–1698.)
- **The Shapiro reaction** (Adlington, R. M., & Barrett, A. G. (1983). Recent applications of the Shapiro reaction. *Accounts of Chemical Research, 16*(2), 55–59.)

SYNTHESIS OF STEROIDS

We begin this chapter with a discussion of steroids (Figure 3.1). These natural products are found in animals, plants, and fungi in which they have important and diverse biological functions. Steroids form the basis for many important pharmaceuticals. Once the potent biological activity of steroid hormones became known in the mid twentieth century, there was a great incentive to synthesize them in the lab. A reliable steroid synthesis would greatly facilitate the development of drugs with a variety of applications. Thus, the pharmaceutical industry was a driving force in the evolution of synthetic strategies that would be of use in this quest. Efforts to develop a synthetic route to the steroids involved the convergence of four active areas of research, namely terpene biosynthesis, reaction mechanisms, stereoselective synthesis, and

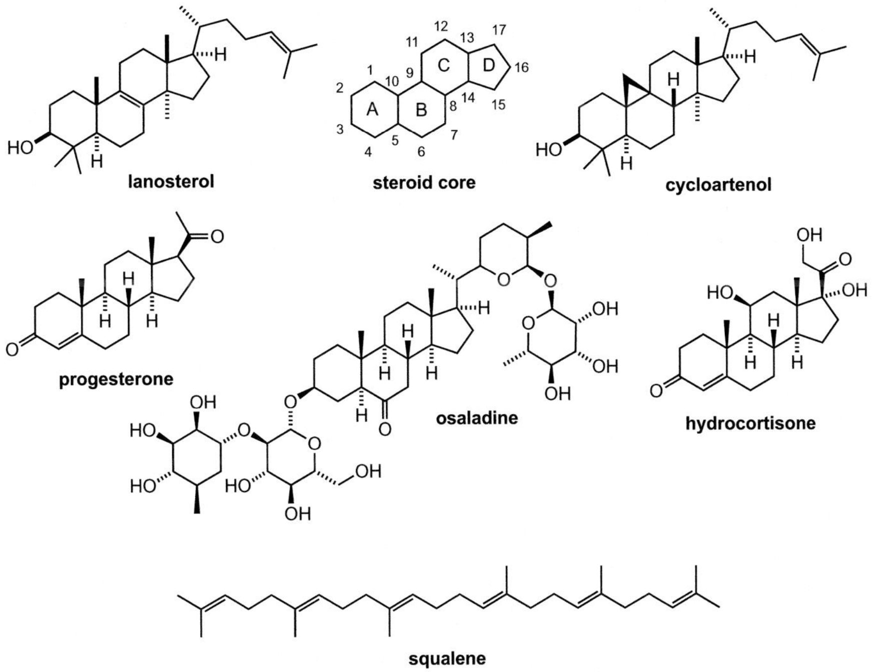

FIGURE 3.1. Examples illustrating the varied structures of the steroids and their biogenetic precursor squalene.

natural product synthesis. This convergence resulted in the field described as "bio-inspired synthesis." The underlying strategy involved building the target structure from simpler precursors following a plan inspired by the enzymatic transformations (hypothesized or experimentally demonstrated) associated with the molecule's biosynthesis. The progesterone story provides the background for this approach.

PROGESTERONE

Progesterone is a steroid hormone that prepares the uterus for implantation of an ovum and helps maintain the placenta throughout the duration of the pregnancy—it is a pregnancy hormone. Agonists of the progesterone receptor prevent ovulation and, thus, are contraceptives. Progesterone first became available in quantity through a relatively inexpensive process that involved the conversion of the plant steroid diosgenin, which could be extracted from cultivated Mexican yams, to progesterone via a chemical sequence that is known as the Marker degradation (Figure 3.2).[1] This is an example of a *semi-synthesis*, wherein a combination of biosynthesis and chemical synthesis is used to assemble the target molecule. Note that all the carbon atoms in progesterone are present in the starting material; no C–C bond formation is necessary. A more economical semi-synthesis of progesterone was developed starting from stigmasterol,[2] a plant steroid obtained in large quantities from soybean oil. This procedure was developed by the notable African-American chemist Percy Julian (Figure 3.3).[3]

As the interest in steroids grew, several academic laboratories were busy trying to reconcile the observed stereospecificity of the enzyme-catalyzed polycyclization of squalene to a variety of triterpenes that included steroids. These investigations led to formulation of what has become known as the Stork–Eschenmoser hypothesis (Figure 3.4A), which, in its essence, states that:

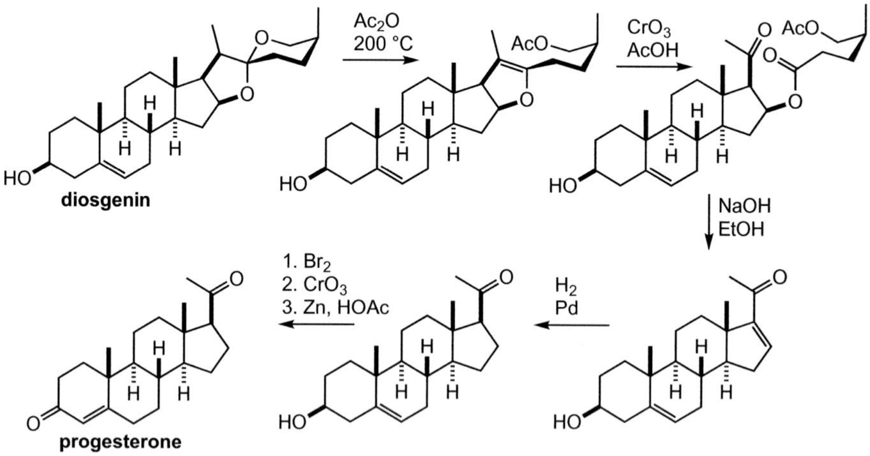

FIGURE 3.2.   The Marker degradation.

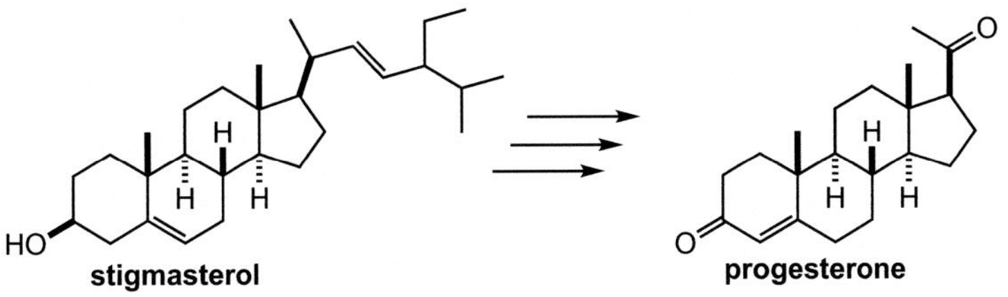

FIGURE 3.3. An alternate source of progesterone.

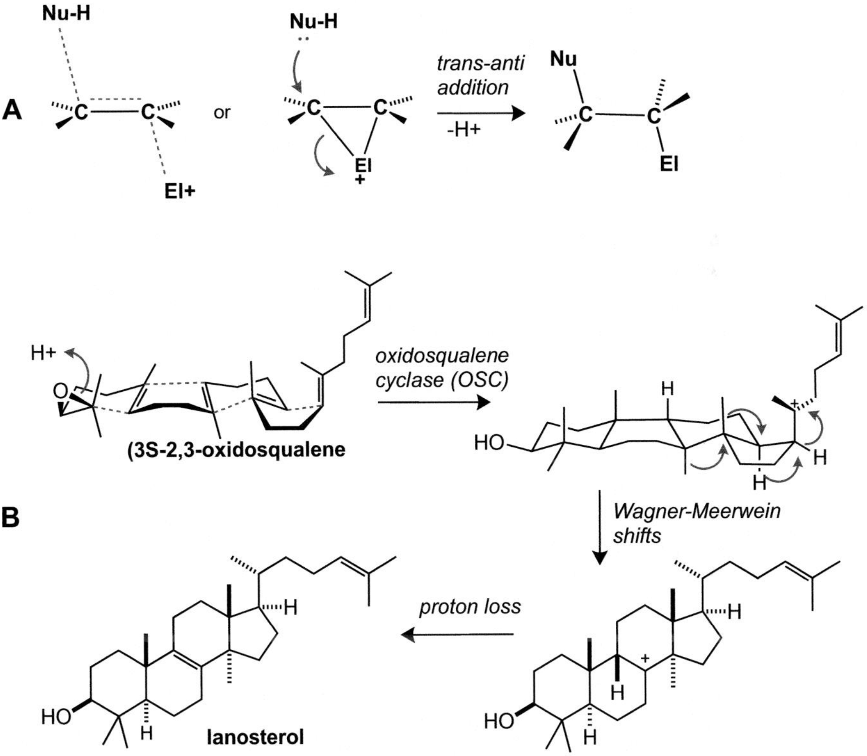

FIGURE 3.4. (A) Essence of the Stork–Eschenmoser hypothesis. (B) The biosynthesis of lanosterol.

when an acid-catalyzed polyene cyclization proceeds under stereoelectronic control (either as a 'concerted' process or, what is stereochemically equivalent, as a stepwise process via carbocationic intermediates that retain stereochemical information), then the stereochemical outcome will correspond to stereospecific trans-additions at C=C bonds.

In other words, the addition of a polarized reagent across a double bond occurs in an anti fashion in order to maximize orbital overlap.[4] The stereochemical information of the alkene (E or Z) is transferred to the configuration of the corresponding sp³ carbon atoms in the product. The overall configuration of a particular product is dependent on the conformation that squalene adopts in the presence of the cyclase. Thus, a chair, boat, chair pre-cyclization conformation leads to the lanosterol ABC ring system. The hypothesis also succeeded in rationalizing the observed stereospecificity of subsequent carbenium ion-initiated domino[5] Wagner–Meerwein rearrangements (which are simply carbenium and/or carbonium ion-mediated 1,2-hydride and 1,2-alkyl shifts)[6] to give the final steroid structure (lanosterol in Figure 3.4B). These studies raised the question: could the Stork–Eschenmoser hypothesis be applied to the chemical synthesis of steroidal hormones?

TOTAL SYNTHESIS OF PROGESTERONE

William S. Johnson's bioinspired progesterone synthesis[7] provided an affirmative answer to this question. The key polycyclization reaction in the synthesis began with the acyclic starting material shown in Figure 3.5. The stereocontrolled synthesis of this compound will be discussed shortly. This polycyclization substrate incorporated a cyclic allylic alcohol as a carbenium precursor and an acetylene as a carbenium terminating group. Exposure of this compound to trifluoroacetic acid resulted in a remarkable series of bond reorganizations that formed the B, C, and D rings of progesterone and correctly installed five contiguous stereocenters in a

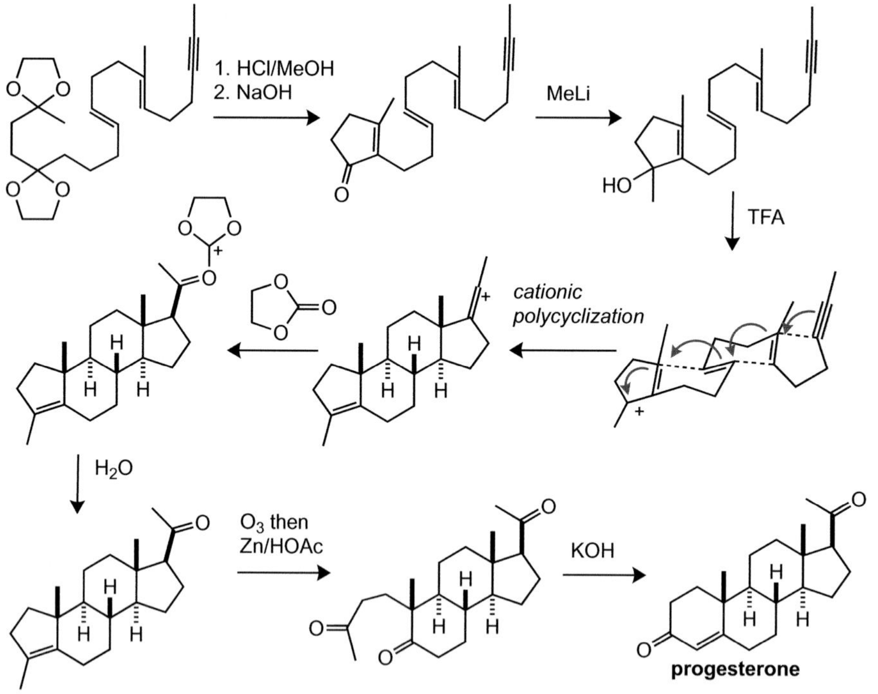

FIGURE 3.5. Johnson's bioinspired synthesis of progesterone.

single step. Ozonolysis of the polycyclization product, followed by an aldol condensation, installed Ring A and completed the synthesis of racemic progesterone in approximately 30% overall yield. Even though Johnson's synthesis produced racemic product, this was a remarkable feat, earning his synthesis a place in the classics category.

In order to set the developing stereocenters correctly during the polycyclization, it was necessary to synthesize the starting dienyne with complete control of the di- and trisubstituted alkene stereochemistry. This is because the polycyclization reaction adheres to the Stork–Eschenmoser hypothesis with the alkene stereochemistry being converted to chiral sp^3 carbon atoms in the product. At the time of this work, the "go to" method for alkene synthesis was the Wittig reaction. Most undergraduate courses in organic chemistry cover the Wittig reaction of "unstabilized" phosphonium ylides, which reliably react with aldehydes to give (Z)-1,2-disubstituted alkenes. On the other hand, the use of phosphonium ylides that are "stabilized" by conjugation to an electron-withdrawing group generally results in the corresponding (E)-isomer. The stereocontrolled synthesis of di- and trisubstituted alkenes that were not conjugated to stabilizing groups was particularly challenging. Johnson's response to these problems is shown in Figure 3.6.

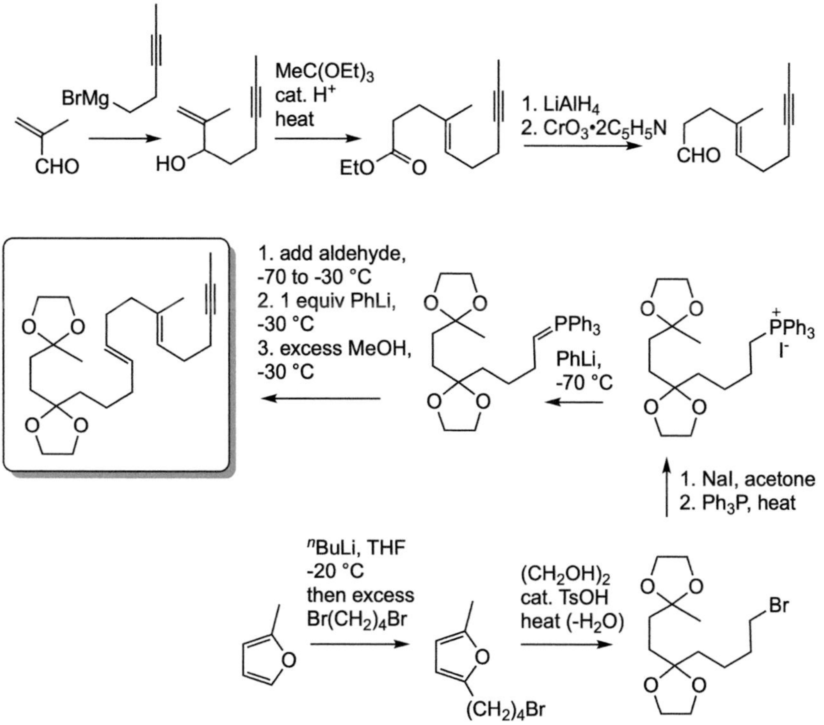

FIGURE 3.6. Johnson's control of alkene stereochemistry in his progesterone synthesis.

Johnson's variant of the Claisen rearrangement, a concerted pericyclic sigma-tropic rearrangement, was used to generate the (E) trisubstituted alkene. The synthetic sequence began with the addition of a Grignard reagent to methalcrolein to give an allylic alcohol. This compound reacted with excess triethyl orthoacetate to give a mixed orthoester intermediate, which upon heating, lost a molecule of ethanol. The resulting intermediate underwent a concerted [3,3]-sigmatropic rearrangement to give the (E)-alkene ester. The (E)-alkene stereochemistry was dictated by the conformation of the cyclic transition state, which prefers to be chair-like with the R group in an equatorial position. This is a pericyclic process that is controlled by frontier molecular orbital considerations. A simple way to see this involves breaking the O3–C4 sigma bond to give two radicals. Actual radicals are not involved; this is just a device that makes the frontier molecular orbitals (FMO) analysis easier. The in-phase combination of the two singly occupied molecular orbitals (SOMOs) occurs in a suprafacial-suprafacial manner, which is geometrically allowed.

Johnson-Claisen Rearrangement

The Schlosser variant of an "unstabilized" Wittig reaction[8] was used to link the initiator and terminal halves together via an (E) 1,2-disubstituted alkene. The phosphonium ylide partner was prepared by a sequence that began with the directed metalation of 2-methylfuran. This reaction may seem counterintuitive because the methyl group could also be deprotonated to give a resonance-stabilized carbanion. Metalation involves initial coordination of lithium to the furan oxygen, which places the anionic butyl group proximal to the vinyl proton facilitating its selective abstraction. The use of excess dibromide ensures that monoalkylation will occur. The alkyl bromide is then converted to the more reactive iodide with a Finkelstein reaction and then on to the phosphonium iodide, which is reacted with phenyllithium to give the ylide. The olefination begins as a normal Wittig reaction, but the initially formed cis-oxaphosphetane is treated with a second equivalent of phenyllithium to generate an equilibrium mixture of α-lithiated betaines that favors the threo diastereomer. This intermediate is then exposed to methanol which forms the trans-oxaphosphetane, producing the (E)-alkene upon warming.

Schlosser-Wittig Reaction

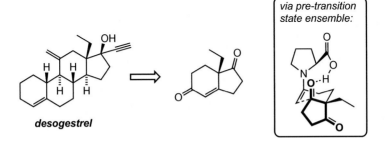

Despite its conceptual elegance, the Johnson bioinspired synthesis could not out-compete the semi-synthetic manufacture of progesterone starting from inexpensive plant sterols. However, the development of commercially viable *de novo* syntheses of steroid analogs continues to attract the attention of chemists. For example, Corey has reported a 15-step synthesis of desogestrel (Figure 3.7), the active component of the third generation birth control pill.[9] The presence of an unnatural angular ethyl group instead of a methyl group at C13 (steroid numbering) increases the potency of the progesterone receptor agonist fiftyfold, but the deep-seated changes in the structure rules out semi-synthesis as an option. The starting hydrindenone is avail-able in enantiomerically pure form via a proline-catalyzed variant of the Robinson annulation (also known as the Hajos–Parrish–Eder–Sauer–Weichert reaction). The

FIGURE 3.7. Synthesis of the contraceptive desogestrel utilizes an enantioselective Robinson annulation that derives its selectivity from a proline-catalyzed aldol addition.

enantioselectivity of this reaction is due to the energetically favored addition of an intermediate proline-derived enamine to the pro-(R) carbonyl of the 2,2-disubstituted 1,3-dione. This is another example of an organocatalyzed reaction (see Jacobsen's reserpine synthesis in the previous chapter).

DAPHNIPHYLLUM ALKALOIDS

An impressive example of bioinspired design of a synthesis comes from Clayton Heathcock's work on the daphniphyllum alkaloids,[10] a natural product family that consists of an extensive collection of structurally intriguing molecules whose bioactivity remains to be fully elucidated. His synthetic planning began with the hypothesis (Figure 3.8) for the biosynthesis of protodaphniphylline starting from an oxidized squalene molecule ($R = CH_2CH_2CH = C(Me)CH_2CH_2CH = CMe_2$). Such oxidations could be performed by cytochrome P450 enzymes. Heathcock had a specific starting material (squalene) and a specific target (protodaphniphylline) in mind, so he simply needed to outline the individual steps that would be needed to link these two structures together.

This hypothesis was experimentally tested by first synthesizing the proposed starting squalene dialdehyde and then subjecting it to mild reaction conditions that were

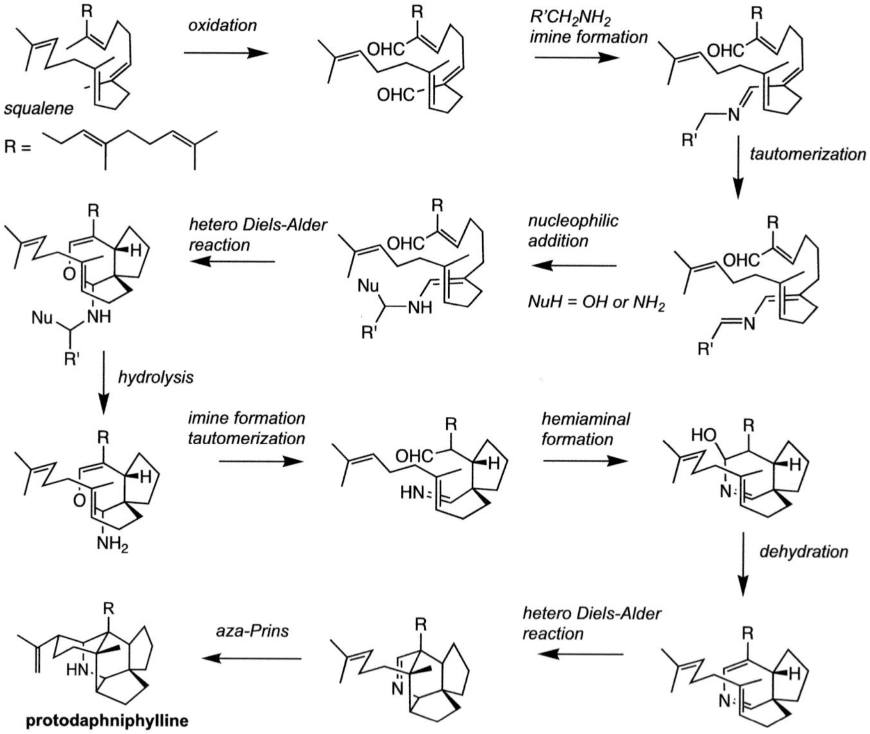

FIGURE 3.8. Heathcock's hypothesis for the biosynthesis of protodaphniphylline.

compatible with the proposed cascade reaction. As is often the case with bioinspired syntheses, preparation of the starting substrate followed a *nonbioinspired* chemical strategy (Figure 3.9). The sequence commenced with the alkylation of *t*-butyl acetate, first with homogeranyl iodide to give *t*-butyl (E,E)-undeca-6,10-dienoate, then in a second step, by alkylation of the derived lithium enolate with dimethyl acetal of 4-bromobutanal. The masked aldehyde was released and reacted with the lithium enolate of previously described dienoate, producing a mixture of aldol diastereomers. This mixture was dehydrated by activation with methanesulfonyl chloride followed

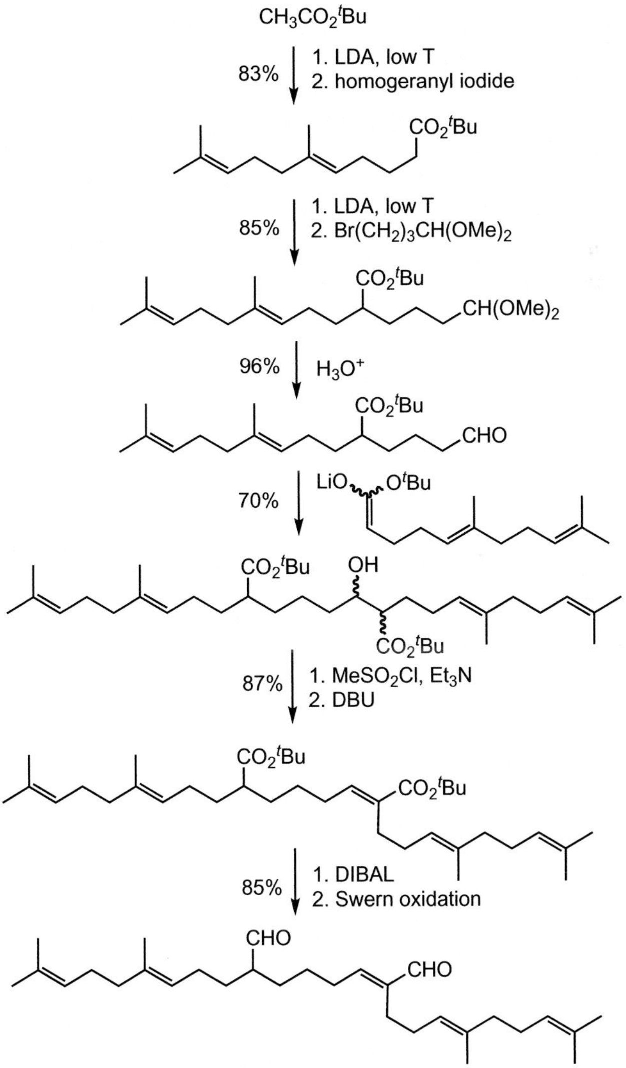

FIGURE 3.9. Synthesis of the (E)-dialdehyde.

by elimination that was promoted by 1,8-diazabicyclo[5.4.0]undec-7-ene (DBU) to give a 9:1 mixture of (E)- and (Z)-enoates. These isomers were separated and converted to the corresponding dialdehydes by reduction of the esters to primary alcohols with diisobutylaluminum hydride (DIBAL), followed by Swern oxidation to the dialdehyde. The biogenesis hypothesis was then evaluated experimentally (Figure 3.10). Treating the (E)-enal sequentially with ammonia and acetic acid resulted in a remarkable series of bond reorganizations that were consistent with the proposed biosynthetic scheme and produced racemic protodaphniphylline in 50% yield. A total of four C–C bonds, two C–N bonds, five fused rings, and eight stereocenters were correctly installed in a single operation employing a simple set of reagents. This nine-step synthesis of protodphniphylline produced a relatively complex molecule in 18% overall yield with a 78% ideality.

A fortuitous incident led to an even more efficient synthesis of diydroprotodaphniphylline when a student borrowed a gas cylinder that contained methylamine that had apparently been mislabeled as ammonia (Figure 3.11). When the polycyclization reaction conditions were repeated using the squalene dialdehyde substrate *but with methylamine in place of ammonia*, a cyclized product that had two additional hydrogen atoms was obtained in 65% yield (averaging >90% per cascade step). The following mechanistic rationale was offered for this unexpected *but welcome* transformation. Rather than eliminate a proton to give a terminal

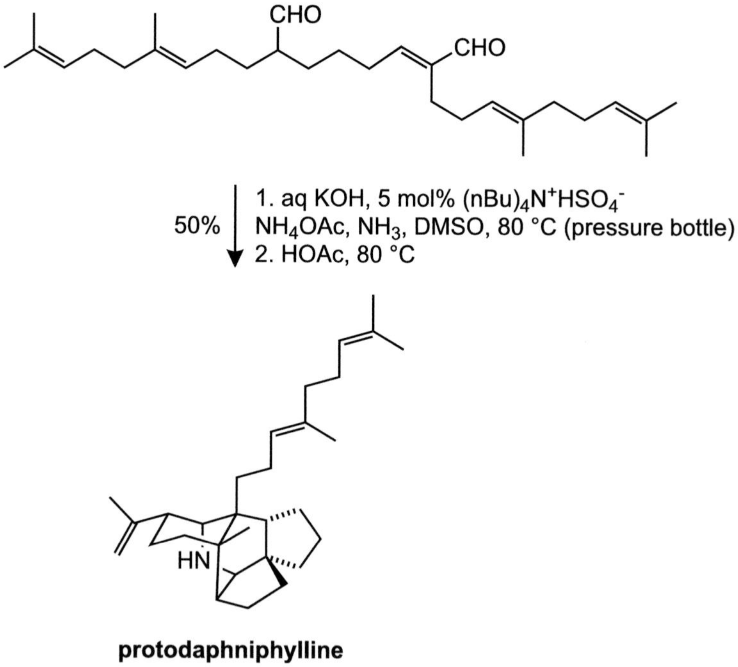

protodaphniphylline

FIGURE 3.10. The key polycyclization reaction in Heathcock's bioinspired synthesis of protodaphniphylline.

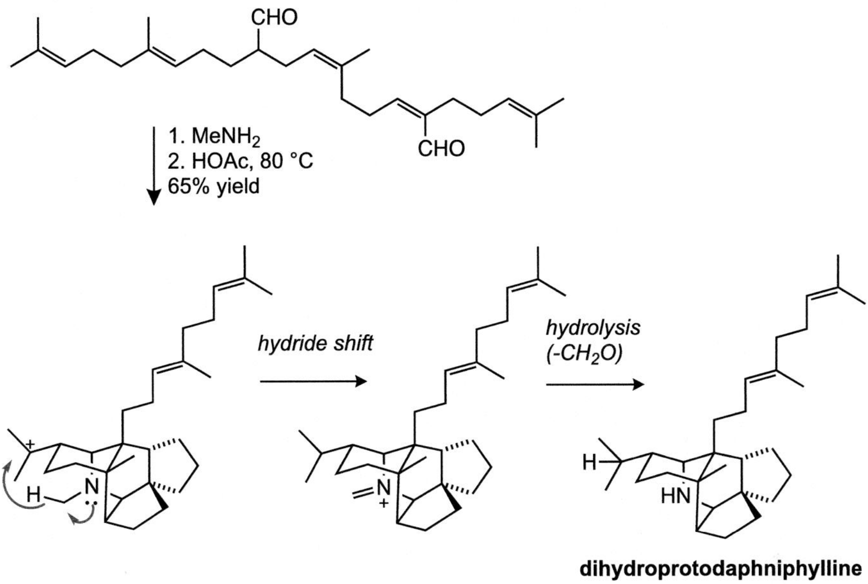

FIGURE 3.11. Heathcock's "fortuitous" synthesis of dihydroprotodaphniphylline.

isopropenyl group, a proximity-induced hydride shift occurred followed by hydrolysis of the iminium ion that was formed to give the observed saturated product.
Heathcock's synthesis of these daphniphyllum alkaloids stands today as one of
the most impressive examples of polyene cyclization and sets a high bar for other
bioinspired syntheses.

PERICYCLIC REACTION CASCADES

The orbital symmetry implications of concerted pericyclic cycloadditions (Diels–
Alder and 1,3-dipolar) were discussed in Chapter 1 using qualitative FMO theory.
We will now add two more pericyclic reactions to the list. Sigmatropic rearrangements are concerted reactions in which an atom or group of atoms migrates from
one end of a conjugated polyene to the other. Electrocyclic reactions are concerted
reactions wherein a conjugated polyene closes upon itself to form a ring. As we
have seen for bioinspired polyene cyclizations, an interesting situation arises when
the polyene folds in on itself placing specific alkenes in an optimal position for
sequential carbenium and carbonium ion-induced C–C bond formation. Similarly,
proximity and stereoelectronic effects can lead to pericyclic reaction cascades.
First proposed for the endiandric acids,[11] such pericyclic cascades can be very
powerful tools for the efficient assembly of natural products. Curiously and unlike
the previous examples presented in this chapter, these natural products are usually isolated as racemates, raising the question as to the role of enzymes in their
biosynthesis.

TRAUNER'S SYNTHESIS OF PF-1018

A recent application of a pericyclic reaction cascade comes from the Trauner lab's bio-inspired synthesis of the natural product PF-1018,[12] a fungal metabolite from *Humicola sp. 1018* that exhibits insecticidal activity. However, synthetic chemists were drawn to this molecule not because of its activity but, rather, for its interesting structure which contains a recognizable Diels–Alder retron. The key pericyclic disconnections believed to be involved in the biosynthesis of this natural product are shown retrospectively in Figure 3.12 with the retrons colored magenta. Unlike other natural products that arise from pericyclic cascades, PF-1018 is obtained as a single enantiomer, suggesting that a protein is involved in the biosynthesis cascade. In the presence of this presumed synthase, the polyene must adopt a folded conformation that places the diene and dienophile in position for intramolecular cycloaddition and not the conformation that would be needed for the alternative 6π electrocyclization. The Trauner synthesis

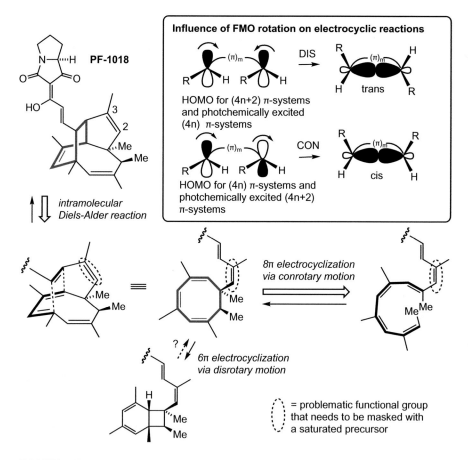

FIGURE 3.12. Key disconnections in Trauner's proposed biosynthesis of PF-1018 (retrons are colored magenta), a potential problem 6π electrocyclization, and the influence of FMOs on electrocyclic reactions.

of PF-1018 is built around this key Diels–Alder retron. An intramolecular Diels–Alder transform leads to a cyclooctatriene, which is the retron for a thermal conrotatory 8π electrocyclization that reveals the starting polyene. In order to avoid the 6π electrocyclization that would be favored in the absence of a Diels–Alder synthase, the trisubstituted C2–C3 alkene was replaced with a differentially protected vicinal diol, which can be removed at a later stage in the synthesis. This temporary structural feature favored a conformation that enabled the desired cycloaddition and could be converted to the target's olefin. The vicinal diol would also make the molecule chiral, potentially enabling the development of an asymmetric synthesis.

Synthesis of the polyene began with Brown's asymmetric allylation of the known dienic aldehyde to give a chiral triene (Figure 3.13). This chiral auxiliary-controlled

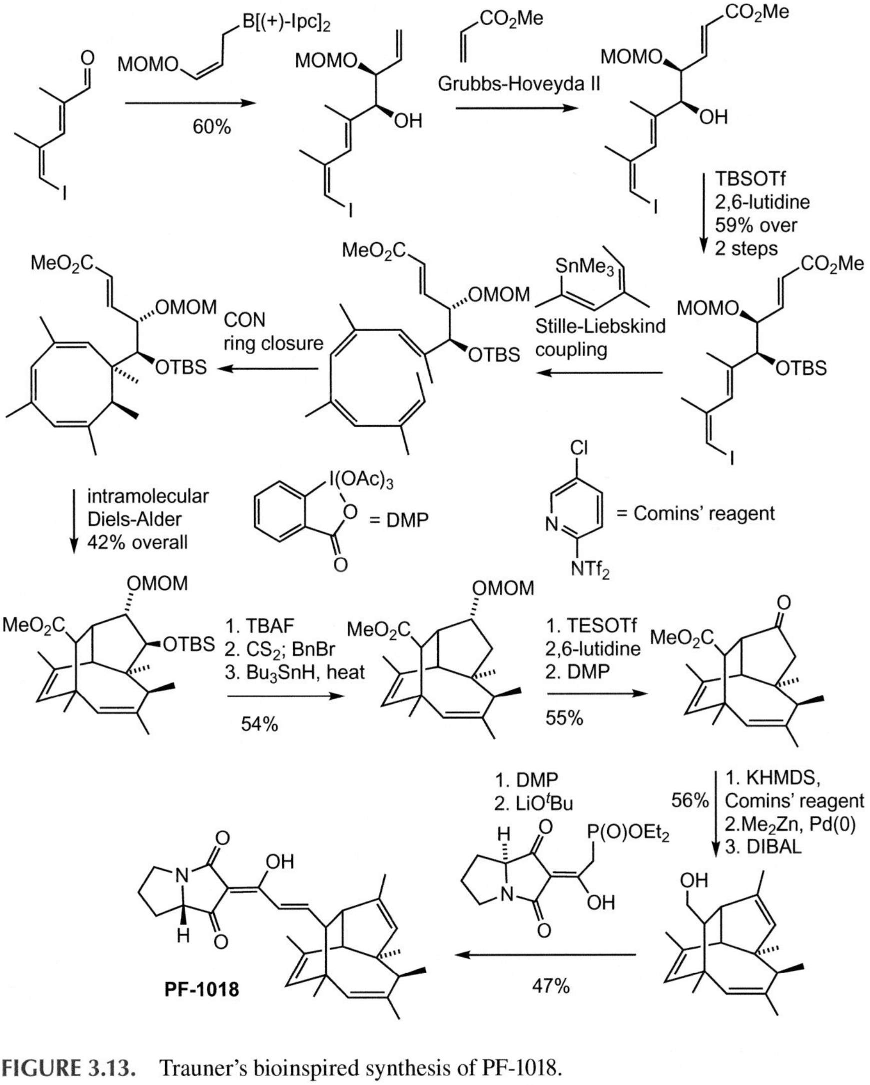

FIGURE 3.13. Trauner's bioinspired synthesis of PF-1018.

reaction presumably proceeded through a chair-like transition state. The observed enantioselectivity results from C–C bond formation on the Si-face of the aldehyde via a transition state that avoids a steric clash between the gauche positioned allylic methylene and the isopinocampheyl methyl group as would occur with allylation on the Re-face. This reaction introduces two new stereocenters that are not present in the target molecule but will influence the chemoselectivities and facial selectivities of the subsequent pericyclic reactions. The triene was then subjected to a cross metathesis reaction with methyl acrylate using the second generation Grubbs–Hoveyda metathesis precatalyst. This alternative to stabilized Wittig reactions was the most efficient way to access the (E)-enoate, as the Brown allylation necessarily produced the terminal olefin. After protection of the free alcohol as its tert-butyldimethylsilyl (TBS) ether, the vinyl iodide was subjected to a Stille–Liebeskind coupling with a known vinyl stannane to produce a stereodefined tetraene that spontaneously underwent a conrotatory electrocyclic reaction followed by an intramolecular, endo selective Diels–Alder reaction to give the core ring system of PF-1018 in 42% overall yield from the trienyl iodide. The structure of this product was confirmed by X-ray crystallography. It was found empirically that the larger the silyl protecting group is, the faster the Diel–Alder cycloaddition is relative to the competing 6π electrocyclic ring closure of the cyclooctatriene system. Transition state (TS) modeling using density functional theory (DFT) shed light on the origin of the observed stereoselectivity. These studies revealed that the two diastereomeric 8π electrocyclization products are nearly isoenergetic. However, the diastereomeric Diels–Alder TSs differ by 6.7 kcal/mol in favor of the observed isomer.

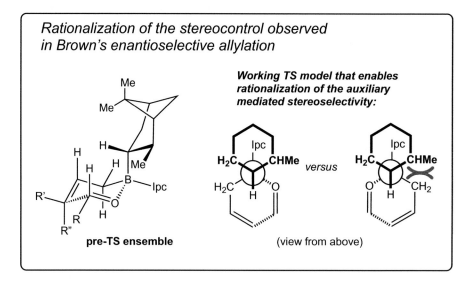

Rationalization of the stereocontrol observed in Brown's enantioselective allylation

Working TS model that enables rationalization of the auxiliary mediated stereoselectivity:

pre-TS ensemble   (view from above)

Rhuthenium-catalyzed cross metathesis reaction

R1
R2
Ru+2
CH2
H2C=
R1
Ru+2
CH2
R2
R1
Ru+2
H2C—CH2
R1
=Ru+2
=CH2
R2
H2C=CH2
N
N
Cl
Ru
Cl
O

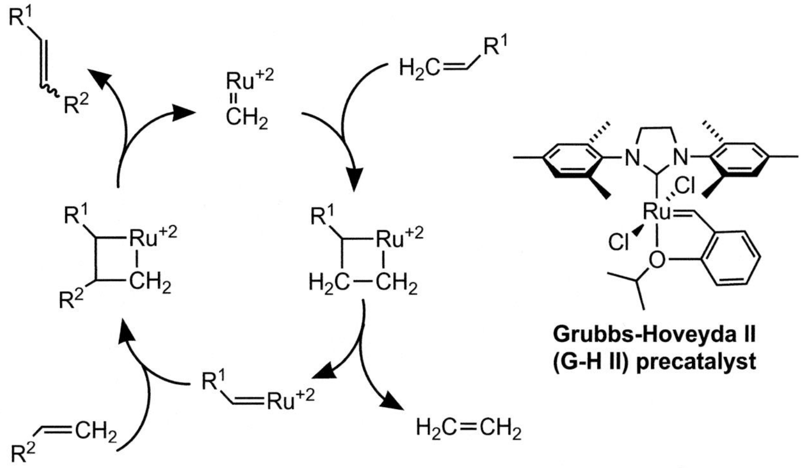

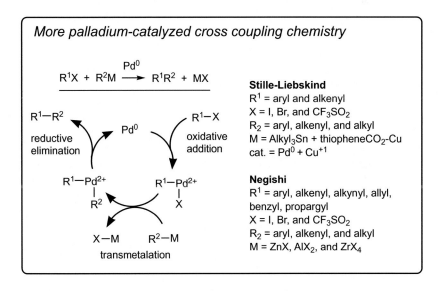

Grubbs-Hoveyda II (G-H II) precatalyst

More palladium-catalyzed cross coupling chemistry

R1X + R2M —Pd0→ R1R2 + MX
R1—R2
reductive elimination
Pd0
R1—X
oxidative addition
R1—Pd2+
R2
R1—Pd2+
X
X—M
R2—M
transmetalation

Stille-Liebskind

R^1 = aryl and alkenyl
X = I, Br, and CF_3SO_2
R_2 = aryl, alkenyl, and alkyl
M = $Alkyl_3Sn$ + thiopheneCO_2-Cu
cat. = $Pd^0 + Cu^{+1}$

Negishi

R^1 = aryl, alkenyl, alkynyl, allyl, benzyl, propargyl
X = I, Br, and CF_3SO_2
R_2 = aryl, alkenyl, and alkyl
M = ZnX, AlX_2, and ZrX_4

Barton-McCombie deoxygenation

The PF-1018 synthetic endgame was carried out as follows. The silyl ether was removed with tetrabutylammonium fluoride (TBAF), and the resulting alcohol was converted to a xanthate ester. The molecule was then subjected to a Barton–McCombie radical-mediated deoxygenation sequence. This reaction began with the generation of an isobutryonitrile radical from azobisisobutyronitrile (AIBN) that produces a tributyltin radical that reacts with the xanthate ester to give $BnSSnBu_3$ plus a thioformyl radical that decomposes to a carbon-centered free radical. This species abstracts a hydrogen atom from the tributyltin hydride generating a tributyltin radical that propagates the radical chain. Unfortunately, standard conditions using a fivefold excess of tin hydride produced a mixture with the major component resulting from the C2 radical adding to the proximal alkene to form a cyclobutene. This result was rather unusual in that trapping of a carbon-centered free radical by reacting with tributylin hydride is usually very fast relative to intramolecular additions. Apparently, the radical is sterically shielded from the tributyl tin reagent. An improved product ratio was seen when excess tin hydride was used, but the percentage of a different byproduct, the C2 methyl ether, began to increase. This problem was solved by substituting a benzyl group for the methyl group in the xanthate and using an excess of tin hydride. The methoxymethyl (MOM) ether was deprotected by treating it with an oxyphilic silylating reagent followed by water to generate a labile hemiacetal that decomposed to the alcohol with the loss of formaldehyde. The resulting alcohol was oxidized to a ketone with the Dess–Martin periodinane (DMP) reagent. This ketone was converted to an enol triflate using Comins' reagent. This is a very useful procedure that converts a ketone into a cross-coupling partner that can undergo oxidative addition to Pd(0). The triflate was then subjected to a palladium-catalyzed Negishi cross-coupling with dimethylzinc to form the trisubstituted olefin.

Finally, the ester was converted to an aldehyde and condensed with an acyltetramic phosphonate dianion to give the target molecule via a reaction that resembles a Horner–Wadsworth–Emmons condensation.

Trauner's enantioselective synthesis of PF-1018 was based on a very reasonable plan that had a biosynthetically inspired pericyclic cascade at its heart. As is often the case with complex molecule synthesis, unexpected problems were encountered along the way but were overcome. The synthesis proceeded in 13 steps from the known dienal and had an ideality of 38%.

TAXOL

We conclude this chapter with a section on the synthesis of Taxol (also known as paclitaxel), a diterpene natural product isolated from various Taxus species (Figure 3.14). Taxol is arguably the most famous example of a natural product that became

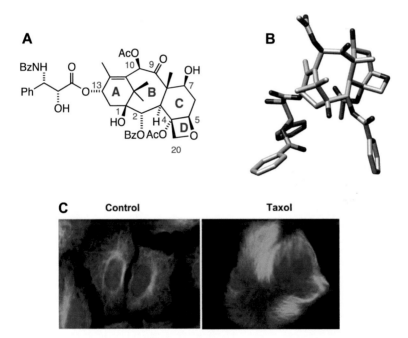

FIGURE 3.14. (A) The 2-D structure of Taxol. (B) The 3-D crystal structure of Taxol. (3-D Image was generated by M. Stone from crystal structure data reported by J. Löwe, H. Li, K. H. Downing, and E. Nogales in the *Journal of Molecular Biology*, 2001, Volume 313, pages 1045–1057.) (C) The effect of Taxol® on the microtubule cytoskeleton (green) in A549 cells. The Taxol treated cell exhibits enhanced microtubule polymerization (right, microtubules colored green), inhibiting mitosis relative to the control cell (left). (Image taken from reference 13.)

a blockbuster drug.[13] It is used today to treat a variety of cancers. Once the National Cancer Institute realized the medicinal potential of this natural product, first isolated unsustainably from the bark of old growth pacific yew trees, a call went for chemists to develop a reliable and environmentally responsible synthesis of this compound. The objective was to secure a supply of the natural product for further testing and clinical trials. Taxol's remarkable antiproliferative activity was traced to its inhibition of microtubule disassembly during mitosis. With the discovery of its biological properties, there began an intense search for an alternate source of Taxol. The resulting world-wide effort crossed discipline lines and included the areas of total chemical synthesis, semi-synthesis, and synthetic biology.

After a heated competition between a number of the premier synthetic labs around the world, the total synthesis of Taxol was reported nearly simultaneously in 1994 by the research groups of Nicolaou[14] and Holton.[15] Depending on where one starts counting steps, both syntheses are on the order of 40 steps in length. An abridged retrospective look at Nicolaou's synthesis is shown in Figure 3.15 using "nested" transforms where possible (the key construction transform is written above the retrosynthesis arrow). Note that most of the synthesis was concerned with construction of the heavily congested core of Taxol, followed by the introduction of ester substituents at C2 and C13. Although the McMurry coupling appeared to be a promising way to generate the B-ring and introduce the oxygen substituents on C9 and C10 in a single operation, this key reaction produced three byproducts in addition to 23% of the desired diol. The synthesis resulted in the production of racemic Taxol that had to be resolved at an advanced stage. Clearly, this total synthesis did not solve the Taxol supply problem.

The Shapiro Reaction

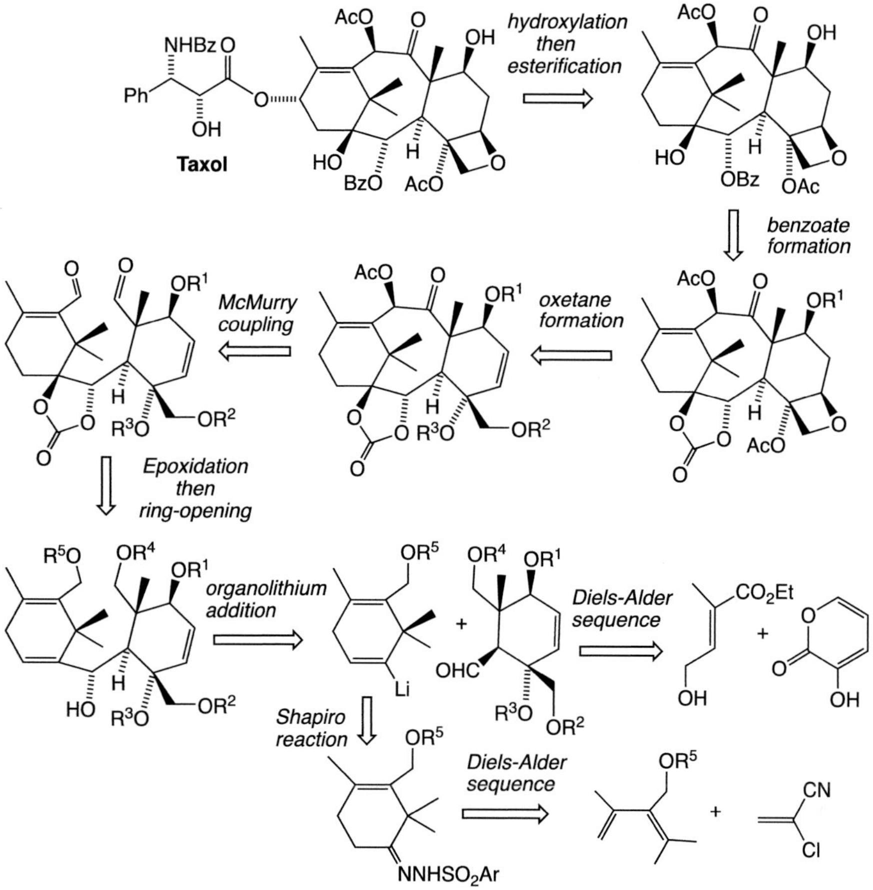

FIGURE 3.15. A condensed retrosynthetic view of Nicolaou's 40-step total synthesis of Taxol showing key transforms.

McMurry coupling mechanism

The supply problem was finally solved by the development of an effective semi-synthesis of Taxol starting from 10-deacetylbaccatin III (Figure 3.16),[16] a compound that was readily obtained from the leaves of a shrub that could be sustainably harvested. This four-step semi-synthesis of Taxol that was developed by Holton began with protection of the most reactive C7 hydroxyl group as a triethylsilyl (TES) ether. This was followed by acetylation of the C10 hydroxyl group. The remaining free C13 hydroxyl group was acylated with Ojima's activated β-lactam to introduce the β-aminoester sidechain (which is necessary for bioactivity). The relative reactivities of the three secondary alcohols in 10-deacetylbaccatin III can be rationalized by their differential steric hindrance (see three-dimensional (3-D) structure in Figure 3.13). Finally, removal of the two acid-labile protecting groups produced Taxol in 80% overall yield.

More recently, Phil Baran's group has explored a bioinspired strategy for the synthesis of taxanes. Because nature makes terpenoid natural products in two stages, he began with a "cyclase stage" that produced the core skeleton of Taxol in a highly reduced form. This was followed by an "oxidation stage" that put the finishing touches on the molecule. These two stages mimic the biosynthesis pathway which uses enzymes to first assemble the polycyclic hydrocarbon ring system of Taxol then introduces oxygen atoms to specific carbon atoms in this core structure. (The enzymatic oxidation of lipophilic molecules to make them more water-soluble is a tactic used to eliminate waste products and toxins from our bodies.) Baran has successfully used this strategy to synthesize a variety of terpene natural products and has sought to apply this approach to the taxanes. A retrosynthetic view of the cyclase phase of his group's synthesis of Taxol is shown in Figure 3.17.[17] Baran's retrosynthetic logic is built on the use of four key transforms (retrons are colored magenta). Clearly, the chemistry does not actually follow the biosynthetic path to Taxol, which involves the

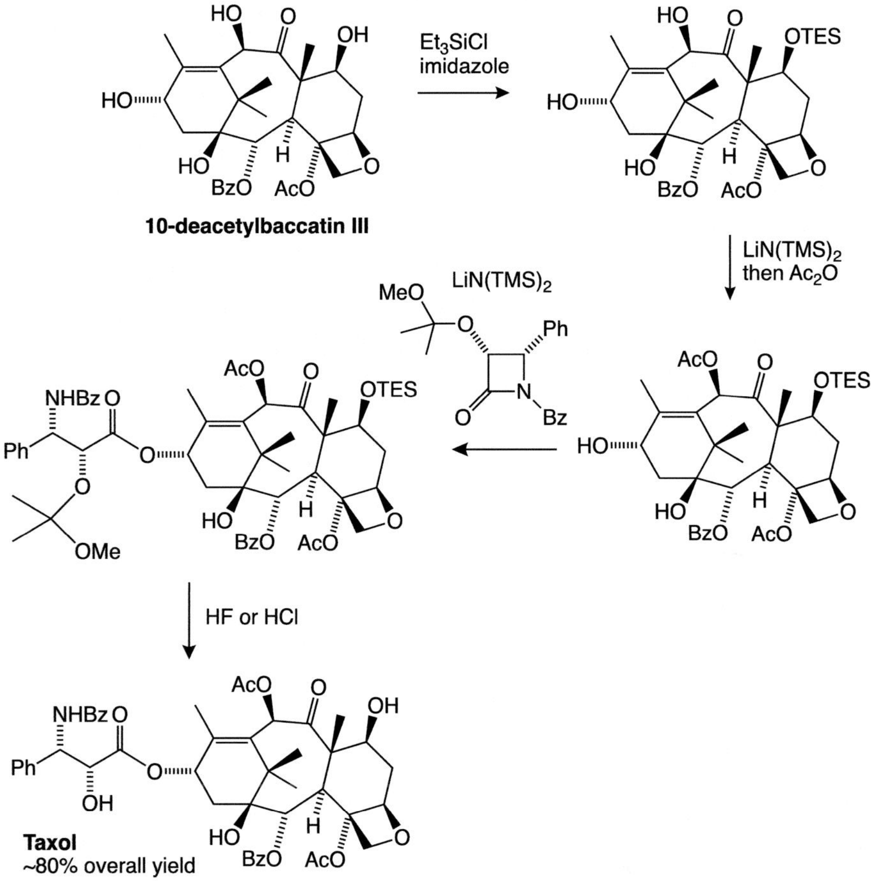

FIGURE 3.16.   Holton's semi-synthesis of Taxol from 10-deacetylbaccatin III.

sequential enzyme-directed cyclization of geranylgeranyl diphosphate.[18] Chirality is introduced via an enantioselective conjugate addition that installs the C8 methyl group. This is followed by a Mukaiyama aldol reaction of the intermediate silyl enol ether and acrolein that gives a 2:1 mixture of alcohol diastereomers. Jones oxidation produced the enone dienophile that underwent smooth intramolecular Diels–Alder cycloaddition.

SIDEBAR: INTRAMOLECULAR REACTIONS

Both Baran's synthesis of the Taxol ABC ring system (cyclase phase) and Trauner's pericyclic cascade path to PF-1018 incorporated intramolecular Diels–Alder reactions. Intramolecular reactions involve the connection of two reacting functional groups by a molecular tether, thus rendering a bimolecular reaction unimolecular. There are distinct advantages associated with such a modification. Let's look at the

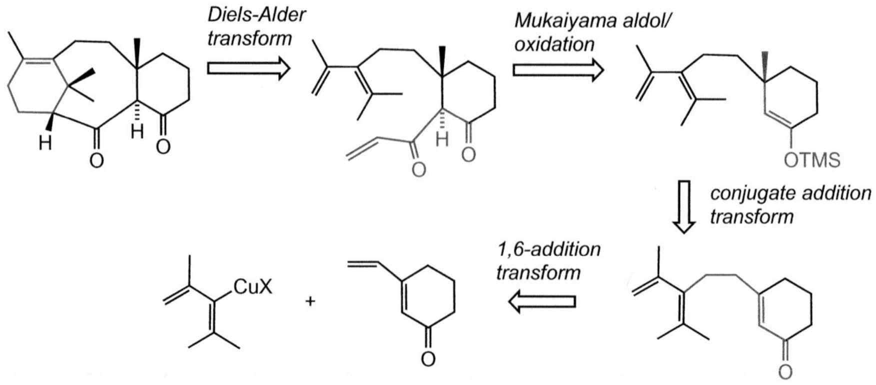

FIGURE 3.17.   Key cyclase transforms in Baran's synthesis of Taxol.

Baran example more closely. First, the obvious: by making the Diels–Alder reaction unimolecular, the cyclization necessarily creates another ring—in this case, the B-ring of Taxol. Thus, if the intramolecular cycloaddition is cleverly designed, the tether can become part of the target structure. This is the most efficient use of the connecting tether. The tether may also be temporary, as it can be removed post-cycloaddition. The incorporation of a tether can have a dramatic effect on the rate of the reaction.[19] To see the effect of the tether on a reaction rate, let's look at a series of Diels–Alder reactions between inactivated dienes and dienophiles (reaction rate is inversely proportional to the free energy of activation). As expected, the reaction shown in Equation 1 is extremely slow. The reaction shown in Equation 2 produced the cycloadduct in a modest 4% yield after 90 hours at 162 °C. In contrast to this observation, the reaction shown in Equation 4 proceeded to give 100% of cycloadduct after two weeks at ambient temperature. It does this by lowering the free energy of activation relative to the corresponding bimolecular reaction (compare Equations 1 and 2). Further rate enhancements are possible if one incorporates rings and substituents to the tether (compare Equation 2 with Equations 3 and 4). One may also apply the "intramolecular tactic" to other reactions, as we shall see in Chapters 4 and 5.

Effect of tether on rate of Diels-Alder reaction

(1) $\Delta G^{\ddagger} = 35.2$ kcal/mol

(2) $\Delta G^{\ddagger} = 29.2$ kcal/mol

(3) $\Delta G^{\ddagger} = 26.9$ kcal/mol

(4) $\Delta G^{\ddagger} = 24.9$ kcal/mol

Although the cyclase phase of Baran's Taxol synthesis was amenable to an efficient transform-based strategy, the oxidase phase was not so accommodating. The regio- and stereocontrolled introduction of oxygen atoms turned out to be remarkably substrate and reagent dependent (Figure 3.18). This, in turn, placed restrictions on the order in which the oxidations were carried out. Many roadblocks were encountered and clever solutions to these problems were developed.

The oxidase sequence began with the use of a Cr(V)-based reagent to selectively introduce the C13 ketone. This mild oxidant was necessary to avoid the oxidative cleavage of the 11,12-alkene that was observed with stronger Cr(VI)-based reagents. This reaction was followed by the selective bromination at C5. Note that the two-dimensional (2-D) structure is misleading, as it seems as though the reaction proceeded through the more basic 4,5-enolate over that formed from the 1,3-diketone (pKa ~12). However, examination of a 3-D model reveals that the C2 and C4 carbonyl groups are essentially perpendicular to each other and, thus, do not benefit from the mutual electron delocalization that would result from deprotonation of a typical 1,3-diketone. The introduction of an axial bromine atom at C5 (a consequence of the α-haloketone effect) apparently induces a conformational change that favors hydrogen extraction at C10 during its radical bromination with N-bromosuccinimide (NBS). While the first three reactions of the oxidase phase each involved the sequential oxidation of a given scaffold atom (C13, C5, and C10), six ancillary reactions were needed to set up the oxidation of C1. This was followed by five ancillary reactions to set up the oxidation of C7, four ancillary reactions to set up the oxidation of C4 and C20, and five ancillary reactions to set up the oxidation

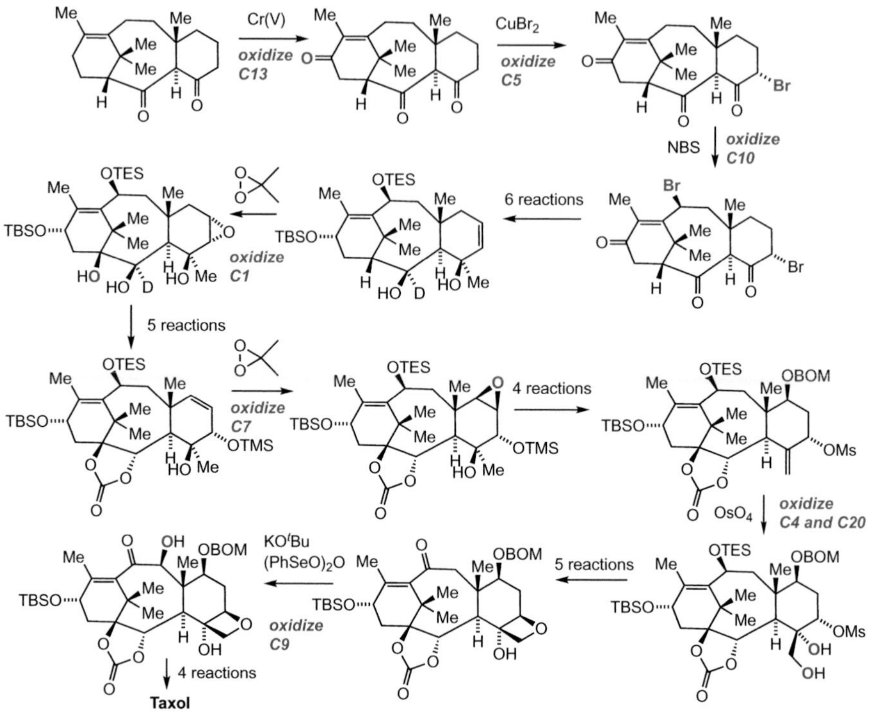

FIGURE 3.18.   Oxidase phase of Baran's Taxol synthesis.

of C9. The two-phase synthesis of Taxol was accomplished in 30-plus linear steps from 2,3-dimethyl-2-butene. Once again, there was no material advantage to this bioinspired synthesis of Taxol over semi-synthetic or synthetic biological approaches to the natural product. Today, the supply line Taxol is prepared on an industrial scale by plant cell fermentation.

SUMMARY

This chapter focused on bioinspired strategies for the synthesis of structurally complex molecules (progesterone, protodaphniphylline, PF-1018, and Taxol). Bioinspired reaction cascades, in which multiple bonds are formed in a single reaction are highly valued in organic synthesis. The examples presented illustrate both the power and limitations of incorporating bioinspired strategies into a synthesis. However, efficiency should be measured for the synthesis in its totality, as the multistep synthesis of a key substrate often detracts from an efficient bioinspired reaction cascade. The Baran synthesis of Taxol illustrates this point in that the cyclase phase was more efficient than the oxidase phase. This work also illustrated the value of a well-stocked reaction toolbox that provided a variety of mechanistically distinct reactions to circumvent an empirical experimental roadblocks encountered during the synthesis.

On the other hand, the incorporation of biosynthetic considerations into the planning of a synthesis can reveal novel reaction pathways to be explored and can result in effective syntheses of bioactive analogues. The value of semi-synthesis for the commercial-scale production of structurally complex natural products is also discussed in the context of steroids and Taxol.

Even though semi-synthesis can jump-start a synthetic plan, native biosynthetic machinery cannot always be used to make unnatural analogues that have desirable properties (making the case for more efficient total syntheses). The growing field of synthetic biology may overcome this problem in the future.[20] From the chemistry perspective, synthetic biology involves reconfiguring natural biosynthetic machinery at the genetic level (gene editing and expression) to make molecules that incorporate unnatural structural motifs. One can expect a quantum leap in the field of synthesis when this technology becomes routine and chemistry and biology work together to create new substances that benefit mankind.

TUTORIAL: RETROSYNTHETIC ANALYSIS OF SALVINORIN A

The Diels–Alder reaction played a critical role in the syntheses of the targets discussed in this chapter as well as the Woodward reserpine synthesis that was covered in the preceding chapter. In the context of building complex organic architectures, the Diels–Alder reaction is one of the most important reactions to have in your reaction toolbox. Its value lies in the fact that, in a typical manifestation, the Diels–Alder reaction generates two new sigma bonds and up to four stereocenters in a single stereocontrolled reaction. Intramolecular Diels–Alder reactions generate an additional ring. Thus, the Diels–Alder reaction enables the growth of molecular complexity quickly.

salvinorin A

This short tutorial will show you how to employ a Diels–Alder based strategy to rapidly assemble the psychoactive natural product salvinorin A. This natural product is isolated from the leaves of the Mexican plant *Salvia divinorum*. It has been used by the indigenous people to attain a hallucinogenic spiritual state. Today, it is of interest as a kappa opioid receptor agonist that could lead to the development of analogues to treat pain, depression, and drug addiction. Our approach to planning will be illustrated retrosynthetically following Steps 1–3 of the holistic approach to synthetic planning that was described in Chapter 1. The overall strategy will be

transform based. This tutorial draws on a recent synthesis of salvinorin A that was reported by Metz.[21]

Step 1: Identify functional groups in the target molecule noting if they activate proximal carbon atoms. There is a ketone at C1 with removable protons at both α-positions, an ester that activates C3, a lactone that activates C8, an acetoxy group at C2, and a furan that can activate C12. These functional groups will help prioritize the possible pathways in our developing synthetic tree.

Step 2: Identify patterns that may suggest simplifying disconnections or the use of powerful transforms. If necessary, add functional groups to create powerful retrons. There is a lactone functional group that could be virtually hydrolyzed. However, the lactone—which is part of the target structure—could also serve to protect the C12 alcohol and the carboxylic acid at C8, so we will leave it intact at this point. Is the Diels–Alder retron (a cyclohexene) present in the target? No, there are no Diels–Alder retrons in the target. Are there any positions that could accommodate the introduction of an alkene via enabling (concessionary) transforms that would be part of a six-membered ring, thus creating a Diels–Alder retron? Yes, there are six possible retrons. The associated transforms are evaluated for viability. Note that all the Diels–Alder transforms require enabling transforms.

Transform A places the alkene in the 1,2-position. Application of the Diels–Alder transform produces a triene that is nicely set up for an intramolecular Diels–Alder reaction. An endo approach of the activated dienophile from its Si-face sets three of the six stereocenters correctly. The 1,2-alkene can be converted to the target's acetoxyketone later by cis-hydroxylation, selective acetylation, and oxidation. Epimerization of C2 is possible if necessary. **This transform is viable.**

Transform B has the alkene in the 2,3-position. Application of the Diels–Alder transform leads to the components of a bimolecular reaction. The diene component contains two electron-withdrawing groups, and the dienophile is not activated. Recall that most Diels–Alder reactions involve the combination of an electron-rich diene HOMO (highest occupied molecular orbital) with an electron deficient dienophile LUMO (lowest unoccupied molecular orbital). Endo cycloaddition gives the wrong stereochemistry, but it should be possible to epimerize the C10 hydrogen to give the thermodynamically favored trans-ring junction. This adds steps. The diene also contains a high energy ketene moiety that prefers to undergo (2 + 2) cycloadditions (see Chapter 4). The conversion of the 2,3-alkene to the 2-acetoxy substructure would be cumbersome, involving conjugate addition of hydride followed by enolate oxidation, acetylation, and possibly C2 epimerization. **Based on these considerations, we reject this transform.**

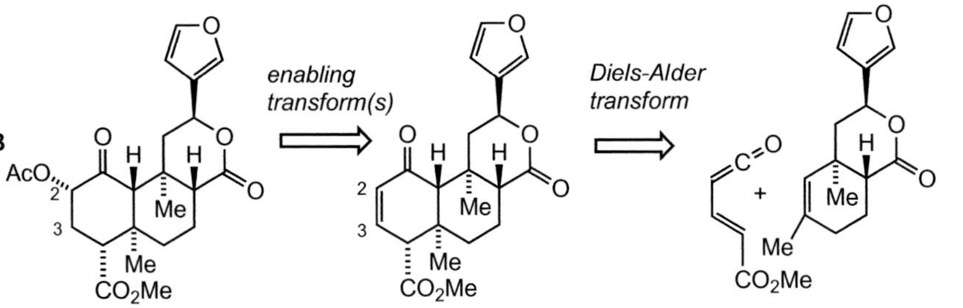

Transform C has the alkene in the 3,4-position. Application of the Diels–Alder transform produces a triene that contains a rather complicated diene with a tetrasubstituted double bond while the dienophile contains a ketene that we have already commented on. If the cycloaddition occurred against the odds, the product's alkene could be saturated by catalytic hydrogenation from the less-hindered β-face. **We reject this transform because the key Diels–Alder reaction is problematic.**

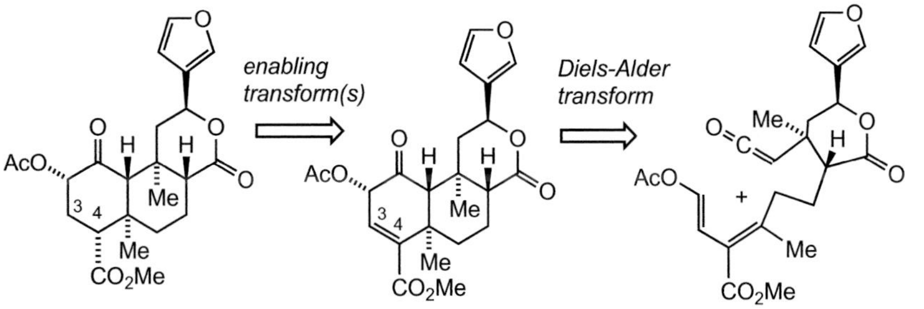

Transform D has the alkene in the 6,7-position. Application of the Diels–Alder transform produces a triene that is part of a macrocyclic lactone. (We shall see in Chapter 5 that this is not a problem.) The result is referred to as a transannular Diels–Alder reaction. The correct stereochemistry will result from one of the two possible exo modes of cycloaddition. The alkene-containing product could be converted to salvinorin A by simple catalytic hydrogenation. **This transform is viable.**

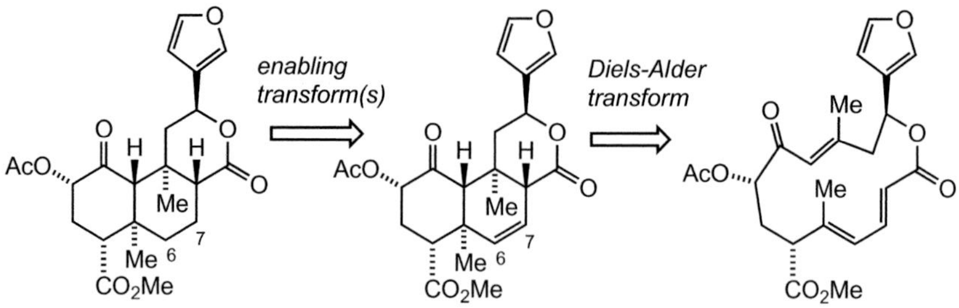

Transform E has the alkene in the 7,8-position. Application of the Diels–Alder transform leads to the components of a bimolecular reaction. The dienophile is some-what complicated. Endo cycloaddition gives the wrong stereochemistry, but it should be possible to epimerize the C10 hydrogen to give the thermodynamically favored trans-ring junction. However, this adds steps. **Based on these considerations, we reject this transform.**

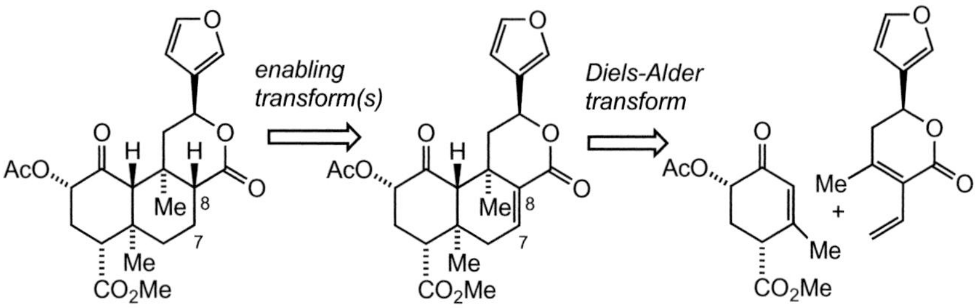

Transform F has the alkene in the 1,10-position. The diene is complicated, and steric repulsion of the acetoxy and methyl groups will not favor the required s-cis conformation. Endo cycloaddition will not give the correct stereochemistry. **Based on these considerations, we reject this transform.**

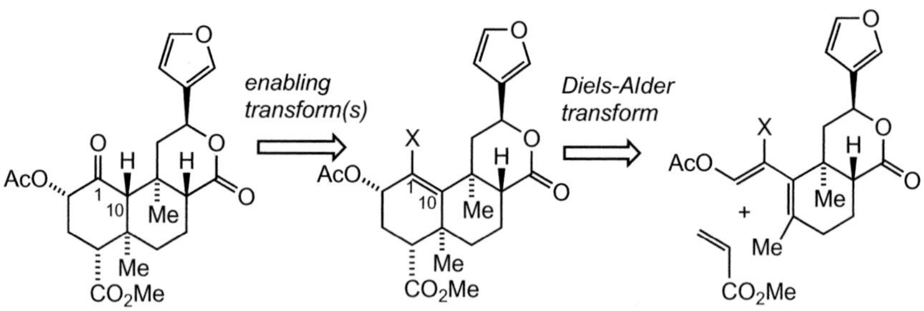

Thus, we are left with transforms A and D being viable.

Step 3: Continue your planning until you reach readily available starting materials.

A synthesis of salvinorin A based on Transform A

By setting the starting triene in Transform A as the most advanced intermediate that we have identified thus far, we can complete the retrosynthetic analysis. First, let's think in more detail about how one might convert the Diels–Alder cycloadduct into salvinorin A. Dihydroxylation of the 1,2-alkene with OsO_4 should occur on the β-face to avoid creating a 1,3-diaxial interaction with the α-methyl at C5. The axial OH at C2 should be more reactive than the equatorial OH at the more hindered C1 position, so Mitsunobu displacement with acetate as the nucleophile will give the equatorial α-acetate at C2. Oxidation of the free alcohol at C1 by any one of the many available reagents (Dess-Martin, cat. Ru(V) + TPAP, Jones, etc.) will give the natural product. The triene substrate will be prepared by reacting the methyl ketone with a stabilized ylide or a Horner–Emmons phosphonate anion. Because a methylene group is not much larger than a methyl group, a mixture of (E)- and -olefins may be formed. The diene can be made by reacting the aldehyde (which should be more reactive than the methyl ketone) with a semi-stabilized phosphonium ylide. This Wittig reaction will likely give a mixture of (E) and (Z) isomers favoring the former, but we will ignore the mixture issue at this stage of the analysis. The ketoaldehyde can be obtained through the oxidative cleavage of a cyclohexene. One might be tempted to use ozonolysis for this reaction, but the furan will also react with this reagent. Therefore, a more selective procedure is proposed consisting of epoxidation (meta-chloroperbenzoic acid (MCPBA) may be used) followed by cleavage by periodate. The cyclohexene is, of course, a retron for the key intramolecular Diels–Alder transform. This leads us to a triene that may be derived from commercially available 3-furfural as shown. Though some potential problems were identified (the synthesis is racemic, the Wittig reactions may not be very selective), this series of transforms constitutes a reasonable initial plan (14 steps, 66% ideality) for the synthesis of salvinorin A and would serve as a basis for further optimization.

REFERENCES

1. Seeman, J. I. (2023). Russell Earl Marker and the beginning of the steroidal pharmaceutical industry. *The Chemical Record*, https://onlinelibrary.wiley.com/doi/pdfdirect/10.1002/tcr.202300048.
2. Sundararaman, P., & Djerassi, C. (1977). A convenient synthesis of progesterone from stigmasterol. *The Journal of Organic Chemistry*, 42(22), 3633–3634.
3. Witkop, B. (1980). Percy Lavon Julian. *Biographical Memoirs*, 52, 223.

4. Eschenmoser, A., & Arigoni, D. (2005). Revisited after 50 years: The 'stereochemical interpretation of the biogenetic isoprene rule for the triterpenes'. *Helvetica Chimica Acta, 88*(12), 3011–3050.
5. Tietze, L. F. (1996). Domino reactions in organic synthesis. *Chemical Reviews, 96*(1), 115–136.
6. Smith, M. B. (2020). *March's advanced organic chemistry: Reactions, mechanisms, and structure.* John Wiley & Sons.
7. Johnson, W. S., Gravestock, M. B., & McCarry, B. E. (1971). Acetylenic bond participation in biogenetic-like olefinic cyclizations. II. Synthesis of dl-progesterone. *Journal of the American Chemical Society, 93*(17), 4332–4334.
8. Wang, Q., Deredas, D., Huynh, C., & Schlosser, M. (2003). Sequestered alkyllithiums: Why phenyllithium alone is suitable for betaine-ylide generation. *Chemistry–A European Journal, 9*(2), 570–574.
9. Corey, E. J., & Huang, A. X. (1999). A short enantioselective total synthesis of the third-generation oral contraceptive desogestrel. *Journal of the American Chemical Society, 121*(4), 710–714.
10. Heathcock, C. H. (1992). The enchanting alkaloids of Yuzuriha. *Angewandte Chemie International Edition in English, 31*(6), 665–681.
11. Bandaranayake, W. M., Banfield, J. E., & Black, D. S. C. (1980). Postulated electrocyclic reactions leading to endiandric acid and related natural products. *Journal of the Chemical Society, Chemical Communications, 19*, 902–903.
12. Quintela-Varela, H., Jamieson, C. S., Shao, Q., Houk, K. N., & Trauner, D. (2020). Bioinspired synthesis of (−)-PF-1018. *Angewandte Chemie International Edition, 59*(13), 5263–5267.
13. Wani, M. C., & Horwitz, S. B. (2014). Nature as a Remarkable Chemist: A personal story of the discovery and development of Taxol®. *Anti-Cancer Drugs, 25*(5), 482.
14. Nicolaou, K. C., Yang, Z., Liu, J. J., Ueno, H., Nantermet, P. G., Guy, R. K., … Sorensen, E. J. (1995). Total synthesis of Taxol. *Nature, 367*(6464), 630–634.
15. (a) Holton, R. A., Somoza, C., Kim, H. B., Liang, F., Biediger, R. J., Boatman, P. D., … Kim, S. (1994). First total synthesis of Taxol. 1. Functionalization of the B ring. *Journal of the American Chemical Society, 116*(4), 1597–1598. (b) Holton, R. A., Kim, H. B., Somoza, C., Liang, F., Biediger, R. J., Boatman, P. D., … Kim, S. (1994). First total synthesis of Taxol. 2. Completion of the C and D rings. *Journal of the American Chemical Society, 116*(4), 1599–1600.
16. Holton, R. A., Biediger, R. J., & Boatman, P. D. (1995). Semisynthesis of Taxol and Taxotere. In *TAXOL®* (pp. 97–121). CRC Press.
17. Kanda, Y., Nakamura, H., Umemiya, S., Puthukanoori, R. K., Murthy Appala, V. R., Gaddamanugu, G. K., … Baran, P. S. (2020). Two-phase synthesis of Taxol. *Journal of the American Chemical Society, 142*(23), 10526–10533.
18. Rohr, J. (1997). Biosynthesis of Taxol. *Angewandte Chemie International Edition in English, 36*(20), 2190–2195.
19. Krenske, E. H., Perry, E. W., Jerome, S. V., Maimone, T. J., Baran, P. S., & Houk, K. N. (2012). Why a proximity-induced Diels–Alder reaction is so fast. *Organic Letters, 14*(12), 3016–3019.
20. Casini, A., Chang, F. Y., Eluere, R., King, A. M., Young, E. M., Dudley, Q. M., … Gordon, D. B. (2018). A pressure test to make 10 molecules in 90 days: External evaluation of methods to engineer biology. *Journal of the American Chemical Society, 140*(12), 4302–4316.
21. Zimdars, P., Wang, Y., & Metz, P. (2021). A protecting-group-free synthesis of (−)-salvinorin A. *Chemistry–A European Journal, 27*(29), 7968–7973.

PRACTICE PROBLEMS

1. What chemical reactions could you use to convert stigmasterol to progesterone?

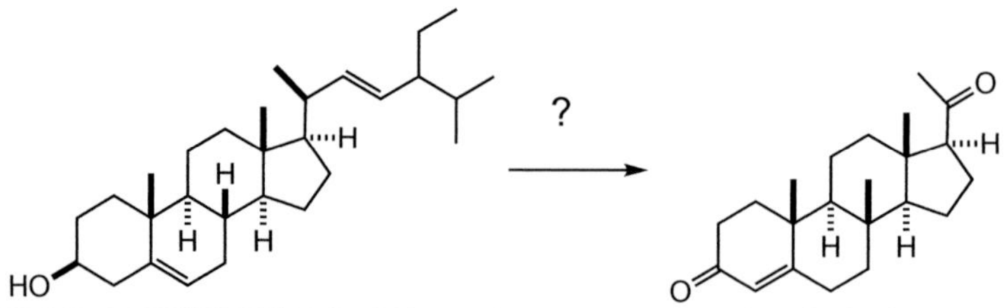

stigmasterol ? → **progesterone**

2. Propose an initial retrosynthetic disconnection for the following molecule.

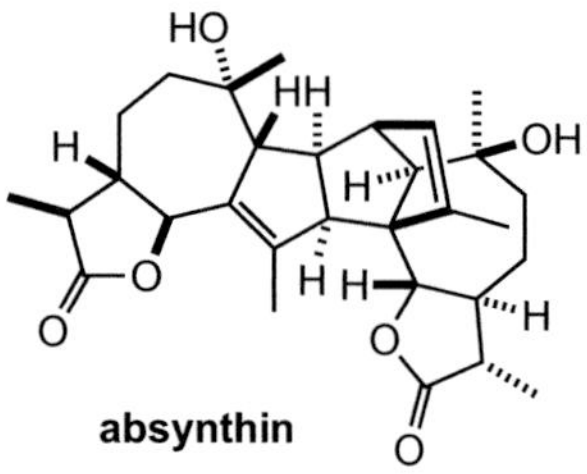

absynthin

3. Propose a stepwise mechanism for the following reaction.

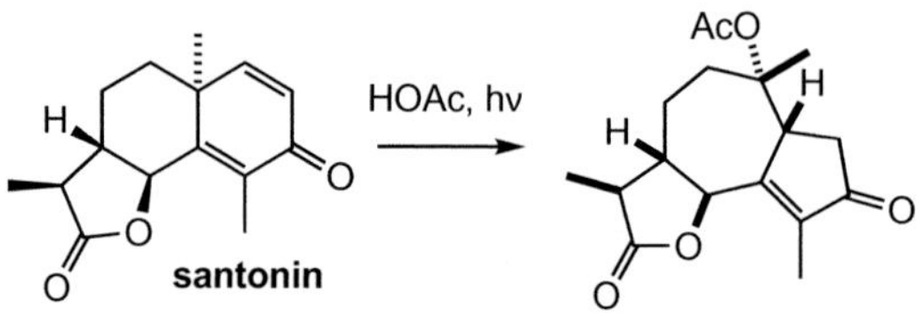

santonin   HOAc, hv   AcO

4. Complete your synthesis of absynthin starting from the product in Problem 3.
5. Propose structures for Compounds **A**, **B**, and **C**.

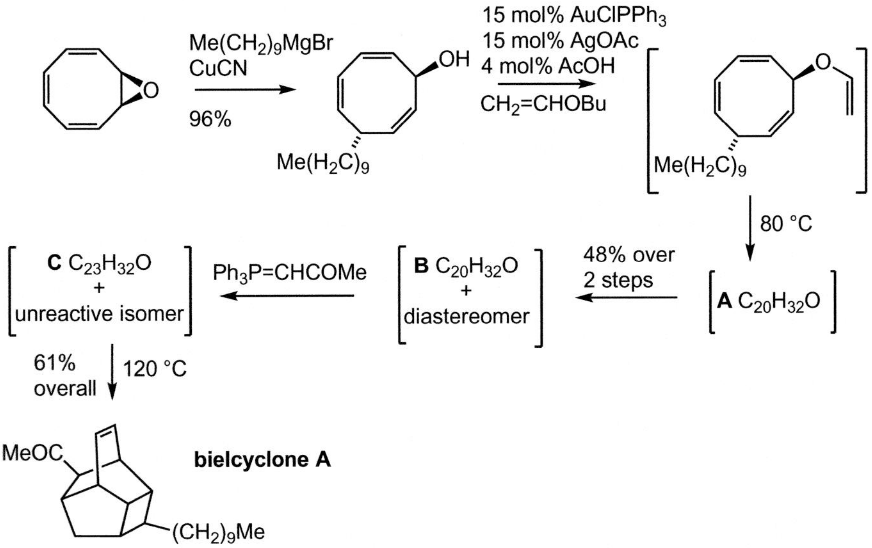

(Yahiaoui, O., Almass, A., & Fallon, T. (2020). Total synthesis of endiandric acid J and beilcyclone A from cyclooctatetraene. *Chemical Science*, *11*(35), 9421–9425.)

6. Show how you could synthesize squalene from succinic dialdehyde.

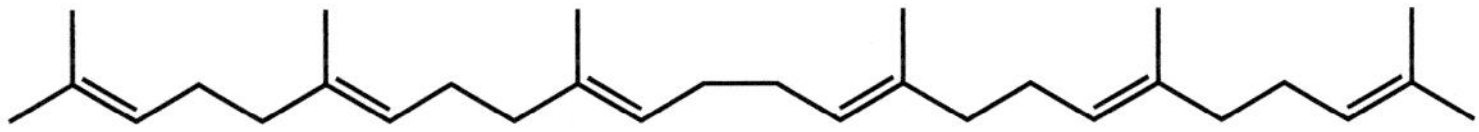

7. Propose a synthesis of salvinorin A based on Transform D.

4 Prostaglandins and Triquinanes

Fertile Ground for Method Development

CONCEPTS AND REACTIONS INTRODUCED IN CHAPTER 4:

- **Catalytic asymmetric Diels–Alder reactions** (Corey, E. J. (2002). Catalytic enantioselective Diels–Alder reactions: methods, mechanistic fundamentals, pathways, and applications. *Angewandte Chemie International Edition*, *41*(10), 1650–1667.)
- **Ketene equivalents as dienophiles** (Aggarwal, V. K., Ali, A., & Coogan, M. P. (1999). The development and use of ketene equivalents in [4+ 2] cycloadditions for organic synthesis. *Tetrahedron*, *55*(2), 293–312.)
- **The Baeyer–Villiger reaction** (Ten Brink, G. J., Arends, I. W. C. E., & Sheldon, R. A. (2004). The Baeyer–Villiger reaction: new developments toward greener procedures. *Chemical Reviews*, *104*(9), 4105–4124.)
- **Radical addition reactions and cascades** (Jasperse, C. P., Curran, D. P., & Fevig, T. L. (1991). Radical reactions in natural product synthesis. *Chemical Reviews*, *91*(6), 1237–1286; Yoshimitsu, T. (2014). Endeavors to access molecular complexity: strategic use of free radicals in natural product synthesis. *The Chemical Record*, *14*(2), 268–279.
- **Gem-disubstituent effect** (Jung, M. E., & Piizzi, G. (2005). Gem-disubstituent effect: theoretical basis and synthetic applications. *Chemical Reviews*, *105*(5), 1735–1766.)
- **The Paternò–Büchi reaction** (Freneau, M., & Hoffmann, N. (2017). The Paternò–Büchi reaction—Mechanisms and application to organic synthesis. *Journal of Photochemistry and Photobiology C: Photochemistry Reviews*, *33*, 83–108.)

PROSTAGLANDINS

The prostaglandins are a family of arachidonic acid metabolites produced in nearly all animal cells that exert potent and varied biological effects that depend on the cell type. As such, the prostaglandins are of great interest in the context of drug development. The 1982 Nobel Prize in Physiology or Medicine was awarded jointly to Bergström, Samuelsson, and Vane for their discoveries concerning "prostaglandins and related biologically active substances." These lipid-like molecules are

 DOI: 10.1201/9781003369431-4

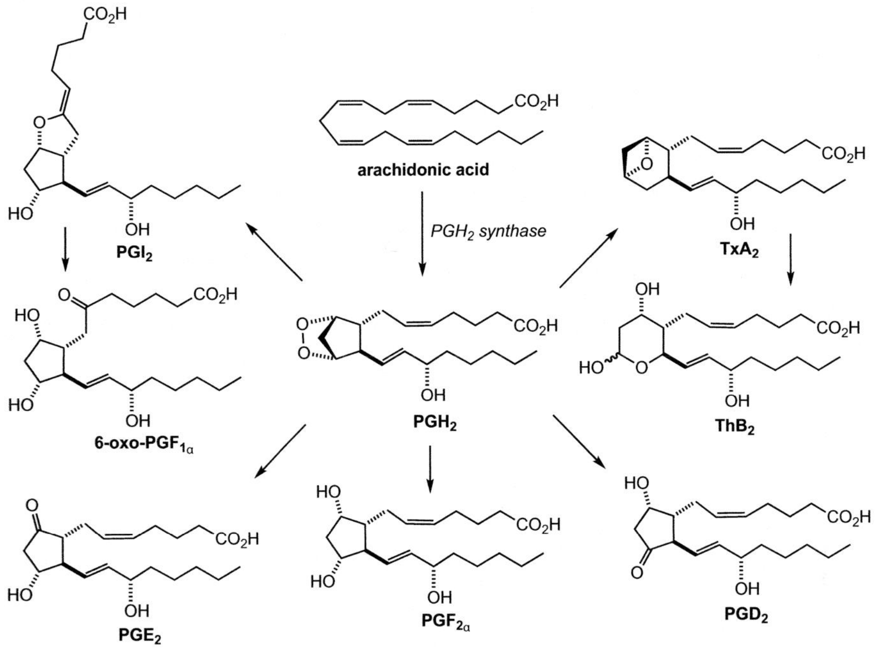

FIGURE 4.1. Biosynthesis of the primary prostaglandins and the related thromboxanes.

biosynthesized (Figure 4.1) from a 20-carbon precursor, arachidonic acid, by way of a common intermediate, PGH_2, that results from the action of a cyclooxygenase enzyme (COX, also known as PGH_2 synthase) on the starting tetraene. This enzyme is the target of aspirin, which is a COX inhibitor. At this point, the biosynthesis branches and the synthesis of specific prostaglandins is completed collectively by the action of cell-specific prostaglandin synthases. Structurally, all prostaglandins are comprised of a tetrasubstituted cyclopentane core that is decorated with oxygen functionality and two sidechains with varying degrees of unsaturation. PGE_2 can be isolated in quantity from sheep seminal vesicles. However, the remaining bioactive prostaglandins are not naturally abundant, making them ideal candidates for chemical synthesis.

PHYSIOLOGICAL EFFECTS OF PROSTAGLANDINS

- Mediate inflammatory response.
- Mediate production of pain and fever.
- Mediate regulation of blood pressure.
- Mediate induction of blood clotting.
- Mediate the induction of labor.
- Mediate the sleep/wake cycle.

SYNTHESIS OF PGF$_{2\alpha}$

- E. J. Corey's lab led the quest for a *de novo* chemical synthesis of prostaglandins, developing useful new chemical methodology along the way.[1] Corey's classic retrosynthetic disconnection of PGF$_{2\alpha}$ is shown in Figure 4.2. This retrospective depiction of the actual synthesis of PGF$_{2\alpha}$ is a useful way to illustrate the retron and transform concepts. The analysis begins with the transform for an unstabilized Wittig reaction that installs the (Z)-disubstituted alkene at the 5–6 position. This is followed by a functional group interconversion that includes a stereocontrolled reduction of the C15 ketone as well as the semi-reduction of a lactone. The enone is the retron for a Horner–Wadsworth–Emmons transform. This leads to a bicyclic lactone aldehyde, often referred to as a "Corey lactone," which is not only a key intermediate in the PGF$_{2\alpha}$ synthesis but can also serve as a starting point for the synthesis of other members of the prostaglandin family. The Corey lactone incorporates the target's core cyclopentane ring with four chemically differentiated substituents attached to stereogenic carbon atoms in the correct prostaglandin configurations. As we shall see, the stereochemistry is a consequence of the stereocontrolled manipulation of a rigid bicyclo[2.2.1]heptane ring system. The C12 aldehyde, a functional group that is expected to readily form an enolate in the presence of

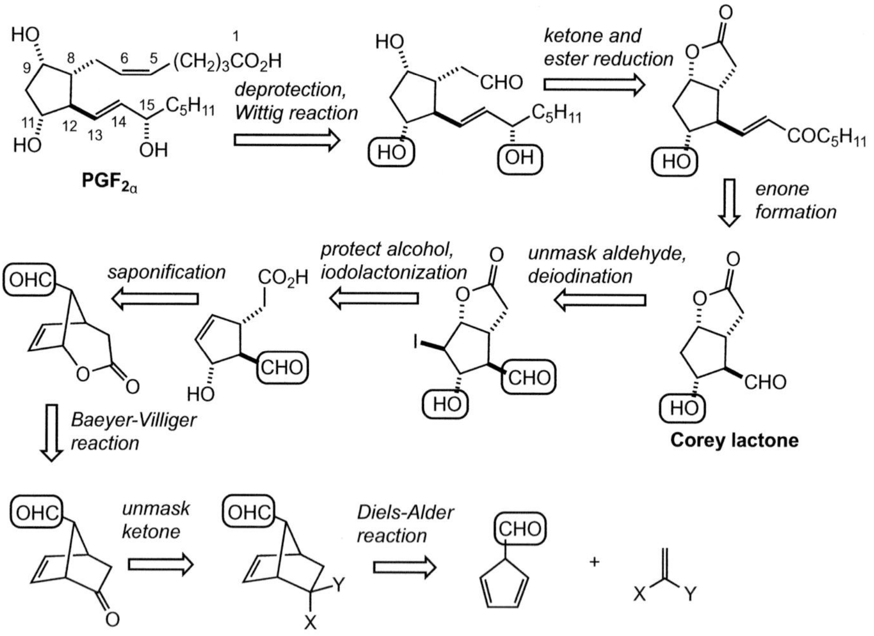

FIGURE 4.2.   Retrosynthetic analysis of Corey's PGF$_{2\alpha}$ synthesis.

base, is configurationally protected, as it likely will prefer to remain anti to the adjacent cyclopentane substituents on thermodynamic grounds if the enolate forms reversibly.

The γ-lactone is produced via an iodolactonization/deiodination sequence on a γ,δ-unsaturated carboxylic acid. Application of a saponification transform results in a bridged bicyclic δ-lactone that is the retron for a Baeyer–Villiger reaction. The resulting 7-substituted norbornenone system can arise from a diastereoselective Diels–Alder cycloaddition between a 5-substituted cyclopentadiene and a ketene equivalent (Figure 4.3). Ketene itself cannot be used as the dienophile because ketenes undergo [2 + 2] rather than [4 + 2] cycloadditions, thus, the need for a synthetic "equivalent." The masked ketene equivalent is usually a 1,1-disubstituted alkene in which the substituents not only activate the dienophile but can also be eliminated after the cycloaddition to reveal the ketone.

The actual synthesis of PGF$_{2\alpha}$ began (Figure 4.4) with the alkylation of cyclopentadienyl anion with methoxymethyl chloride to form the 5-substituted cyclopentadiene. This prochiral diene reacted from its less hindered face with the ketene equivalent α-chloroacrylonitrile in the presence of a Cu(II) Lewis acid to give the endo Diels–Alder cycloadduct. Because it is symmetrical, the use of this diene obviates the regioselectivity issue. The α-chloronitrile was treated with hydroxide to give the substituted norbornenone in a reaction that has been shown to proceed through an α-chloroamide intermediate.[2] This compound was subjected to a Baeyer–Villiger oxidation with m-chloroperbenzoic acid (mCPBA), a reaction in which one of the ketone substituents migrates to the carbonyl oxygen, selectively installing the prostaglandin oxygen atom at C11. In this rearrangement, the nucleophilic peroxycarboxylate first adds to the electrophilic ketone. This sets up a situation in which the more electron-rich ketone substituent can migrate to the electron-deficient oxygen atom via the conformation that maintains a trans-anti relationship between the migrating group and carboxylate leaving group. Although peracids are capable of epoxidizing alkenes such as the norbornene, this potentially competing reaction is generally

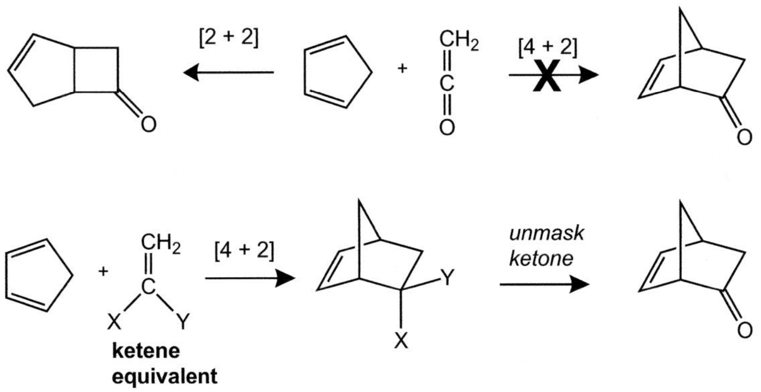

FIGURE 4.3.   The cycloaddition chemistry of ketene and its synthetic equivalents.

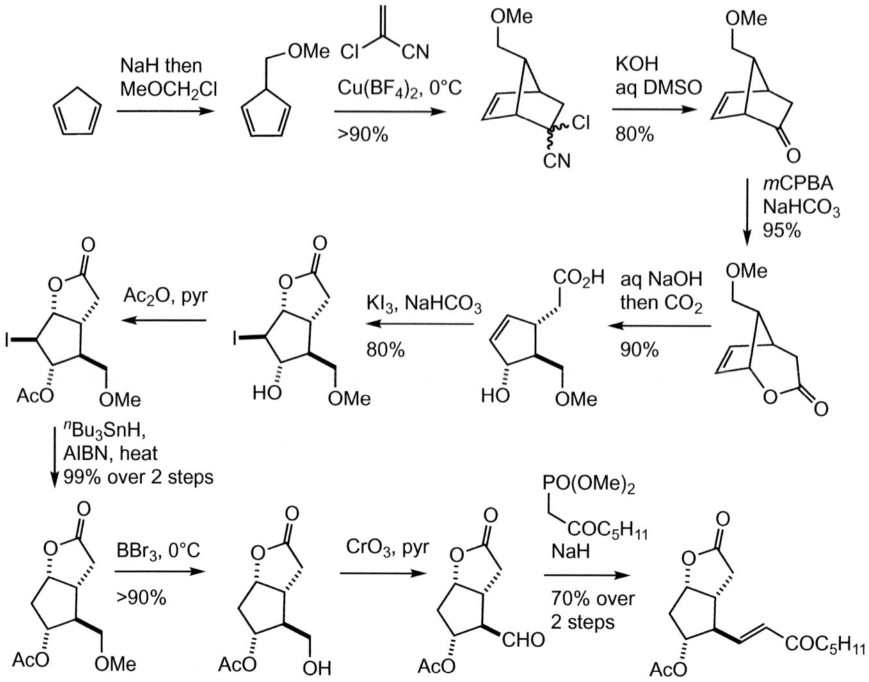

FIGURE 4.4. Synthesis and homologation of the "Corey lactone."

much slower than the desired Baeyer–Villiger rearrangement. Inclusion of bicarbonate in the reaction ensures that acid-catalyzed transesterification won't occur. Saponification of the resulting lactone produced a hydroxy acid that was poised for introduction of oxygen at C9.

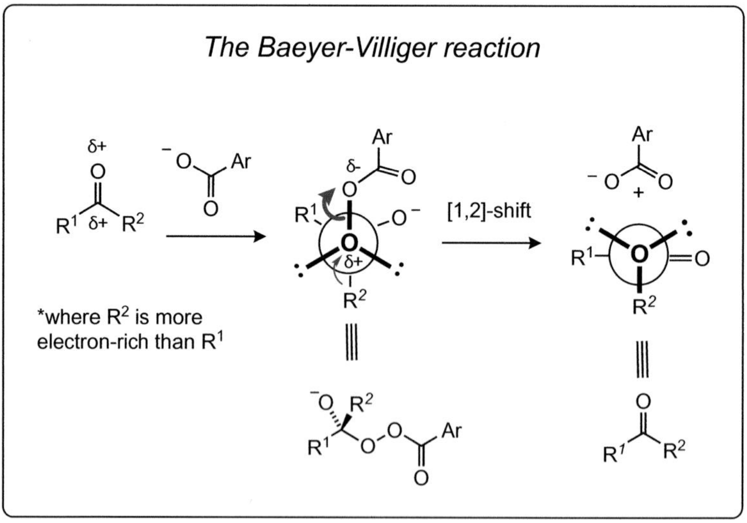

The C9 oxygen atom was introduced via an iodolactonization reaction that involved the ring opening of a transient iodonium intermediate. While iodonium species can form on either olefin face, only the one that can undergo displacement with inversion by the nucleophilic carboxylate is observed. The free C11 alcohol was then protected as an acetate. Note the expediency of using the lactone functional group to simultaneously protect the C9 alcohol and the C6 carboxylic acid that will eventually be converted to an aldehyde. Having served its purpose of activating the olefin for nucleophilic attack, the iodine atom was removed in a radical chain reaction in which the C–I bond was homolytically cleaved to form a carbon-centered radical that reacted with tributyltin hydride. After removal of the methyl ether protecting group with the Lewis acid boron tribromide, the C13 aldehyde was formed by controlled oxidation using chromium trioxide in pyridine (Collins reagent). This oxidation reagent, which stops at the aldehyde stage, is an "older cousin" to pyridinium chlorochromate (PCC), which students may already be familiar with. The newly formed aldehyde was then reacted with a β-ketophosphonate anion under Horner–Emmons–Wadsworth conditions to give the desired (E)-enone.

Diastereoselective reduction of this ketone posed a significant challenge at the time of this synthesis (Figure 4.5). Reduction using the achiral reagent zinc borohydride gave an equimolar mixture of diastereomers showing that the substrate's inherent chirality was not influencing the facial selectivity of the hydride addition. The lack of selectivity in the reduction was partially compensated for, as the undesired 15R diastereomer could be converted back to the ketone and resubjected to the borohydride reduction. At this point, the protecting groups were adjusted. The C11 alcohol was released, and then both alcohols were protected as their tetrahydropyranyl ethers. The decision to use THP protecting groups was governed by the fact that they could be removed under very mild acid conditions at the end of the synthesis.

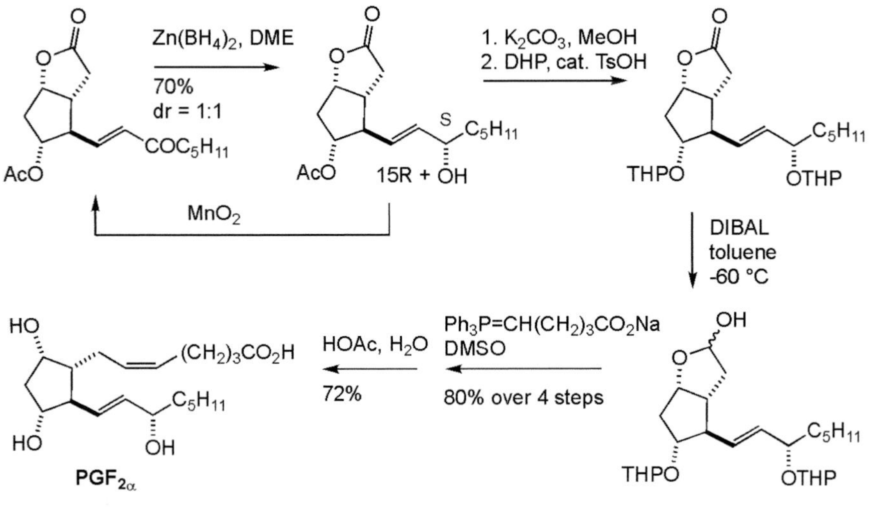

FIGURE 4.5.   Corey's synthetic "end game" for PGF$_{2\alpha}$.

(This was particularly relevant for a projected synthesis of the PGEs that are prone to β -elimination.) Each THP ether formed an inconsequential mixture of acetal diastereomers. The lactone was then converted to a lactol with diisobutylaluminum hydride (DIBAL) under conditions that stabilized the tetrahedral intermediate, thus preventing collapse to a reactive aldehyde and further reduction to a primary alcohol. Upon treatment with a base, the deprotonated lactol underwent ring-chain tautomerization to produce an alkoxy aldehyde *in situ*. This aldehyde reacted with an unstabilized phosphonium ylide to give a (Z)-alkene and complete the $PGF_{2\alpha}$ skeleton. Final removal of the two THP protecting groups under mildly acidic conditions (aqueous acetic acid) afforded $PGF_{2\alpha}$. This synthesis produced racemic $PGF_{2\alpha}$. However, the racemic hydroxyacid precursor to the Corey lactone could be separated into its antipodes by a classical resolution using ephedrine as the resolving agent. The resulting enantiomerically pure hydroxyacid was then carried through the remaining steps of the synthesis to give natural $PGF_{2\alpha}$. It is worth noting that there is some value in carrying out a total synthesis with racemic substrates first, as they are (usually) more accessible. This enables reaction conditions to be optimized without using up precious enantiomerically pure starting material. There is, however, a caveat in that the use of enantiomerically pure reagents or catalysts. (for example, the Sharpless asymmetric epoxidation) will result in diastereomeric transition states with racemic substrates. In this case the stereoselectivity of the reaction could be compromised if the chiral catalyst's sense of stereocontrol is opposed to that of one of the substrate antipodes.

Corey's prostaglandin total syntheses not only provided access to rare natural products with medicinal potential but also served as a catalyst for the development of new synthetic methodology, three examples of which are shown in Figure 4.6. His development of a chiral oxazaborolidine catalyst that enabled enantioselective Diels–Alder reactions[3] and the Corey–Bakshi–Shibata (CBS) catalyst for enantioselective carbonyl reduction[4] represented important methodological advances. Both of these methods take advantage of the Lewis acidity of trivalent boron. The widely used *t*-butyldimethylsilyl ether protecting group was also developed around the same time.[5] Previously, the main use of silyl ethers was to make polyhydroxylated compounds volatile for gas chromatographic analysis. All three of these methodological advances had a prostaglandin connection.

OTHER PROSTAGLANDIN STRATEGIES

While Corey's retrosynthetic analysis of $PGF_{2\alpha}$ synthesis was logical, the disconnections associated with the sequence of transforms employed may not be intuitively obvious to the average junior, senior, or first-year graduate student. However, the disconnections associated with the sequence of reactions shown in Figure 4.7 should be easily visualized by these same students, as they involve the use of reactions that are taught in undergraduate organic chemistry—enolate alkylation and conjugate addition. Also, the strategy leverages the existing stereocenter of the substrate to dictate the relative configurations of subsequently introduced stereocenters. The starting material, γ-hydroxycyclopentenone, is readily available in enantiomerically enriched

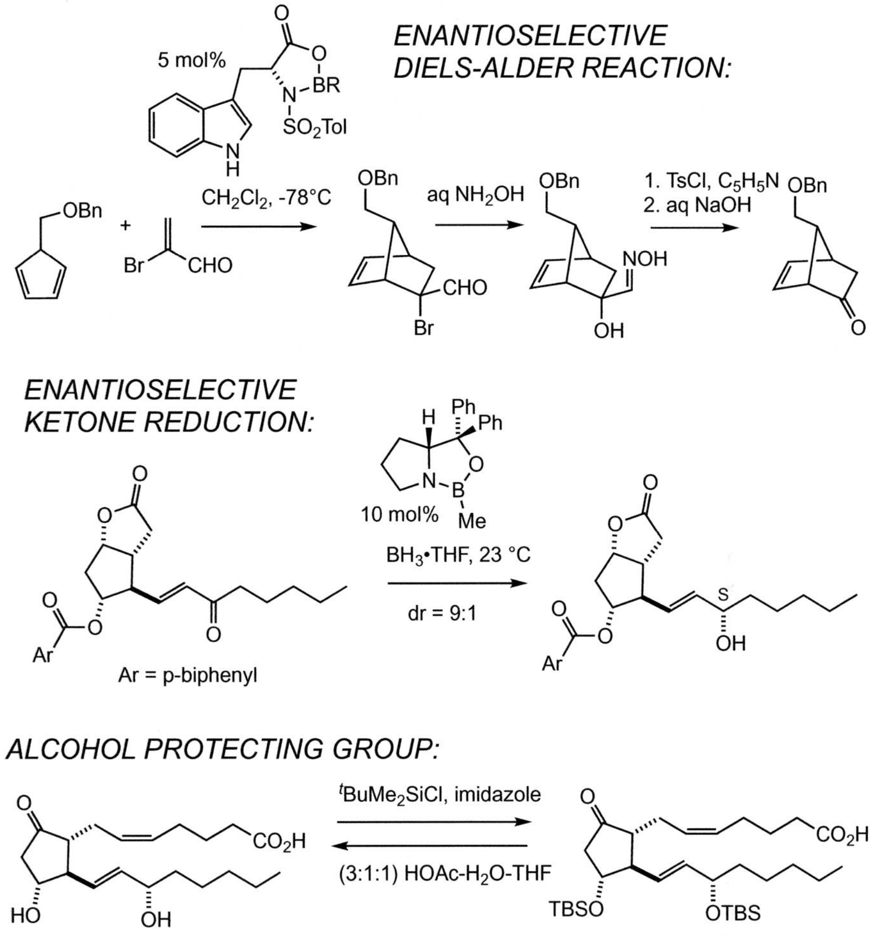

FIGURE 4.6.   Synthetic methodology developed by Corey for prostaglandin synthesis.

form starting from the meso-diacetate via enzymatic hydrolysis of the pro-R acetate. Finally, the plan is simple. These are principles that underlie really good synthetic plans.

However, initial attempts to implement this attractive strategy were unsuccessful. The increased acidity of cyclopentanone (pKa = -log of the acid dissociation constant), which is estimated to be 18.5, leads to the formation of undesired enolates (Figure 4.8), that can produce undesired byproducts. The enolates themselves can also act as bases. Elimination occurs readily when there is an alkoxyl or hydroxyl leaving group in the β position. The resulting double bond can migrate to the thermodynamically preferred position in the ring. Several groups worked to eliminate the undesired reactivity of the enolate formed during the conjugate addition. These

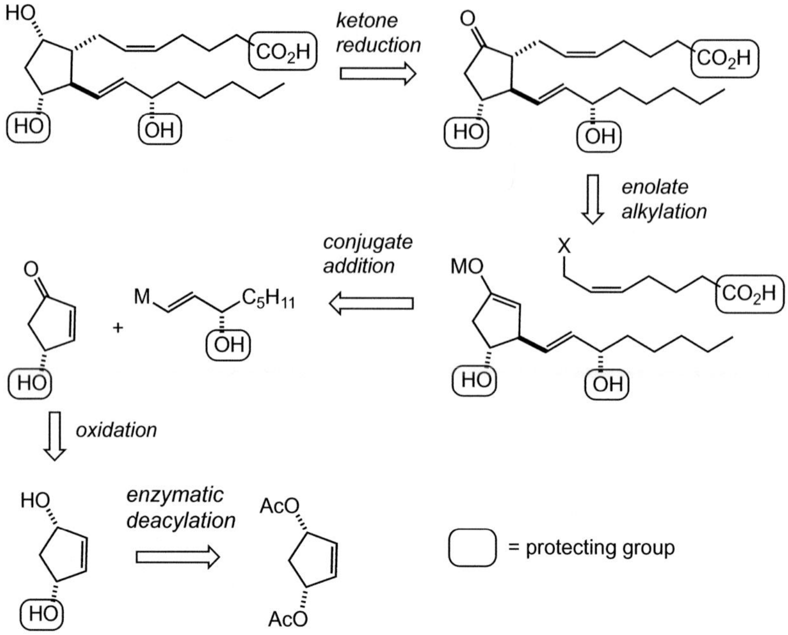

FIGURE 4.7.   Prostaglandin synthesis via a conjugate addition/alkylation strategy.

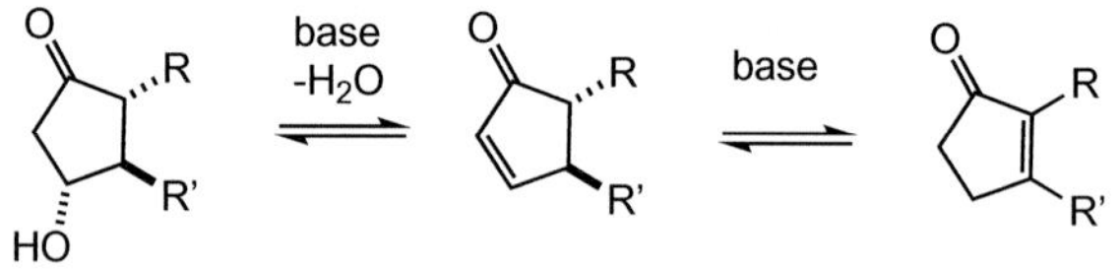

FIGURE 4.8.   Side reactions that are peculiar to functionalized cyclopentanones.

efforts focused on altering the structure (and, therefore, the reactivity) of the enolate intermediate.

Noyori's group in Japan found a practical solution to this problem that involved using a vinyl organozincate for the conjugate addition (Figure 4.9).[6] The resulting enolate species, which is probably associated with more than one metal ion, is apparently less basic and/or less likely to undergo β-elimination. The enolate can, therefore, be trapped with a reactive propargylic iodide to give a PGE_2 precursor in good yield. It will be noticed that tert-butyldimethylsilyl (TBS) ethers were used to protect the alcohols at C11 and C15 instead of THP ethers. Why was this change made? As was mentioned earlier, THP ethers are formed as mixtures of diastereomers at the acetal carbon. This means that a racemic molecule with two THP ethers will be a mixture of 4 (2^2) diastereomers, complicating the purification and characterization of the products. On the other hand, the same molecule with two TBS ethers will be a single species, simplifying its purification and characterization.

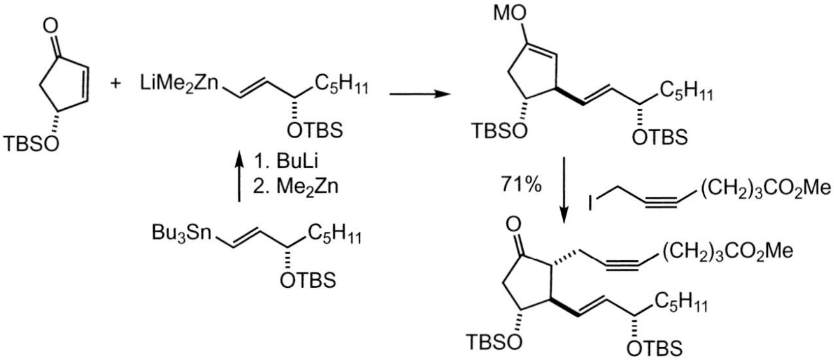

FIGURE 4.9. Noyori's 1-pot synthesis of an advanced prostaglandin intermediate.

A very clever and practical approach to the prostaglandin skeleton was recently disclosed by the Aggarwal group (Figure 4.10).[7] The key retrosynthetic disconnections are shown below. Starting with a compound that resembles one of Corey's advanced prostaglandin intermediates, application of an ozonolysis/reduction transform has the C11 alcohol coming from the oxidative cleavage of the exocyclic trimethylsilyl enol ether. This transform was linked to the conjugate addition reaction. Application of an acetal forming transform produces a structure that can arise from the interaction of two succinaldehyde molecules as shown.

Aggarwal realized that the initial aldol addition could be made enantioselective by using (S)-proline as a catalyst (Figure 4.11). The resulting enantioselective organocatalytic reaction (a relative of the original Hajos–Parrish–Eder–Sauer–Weichert reaction) had been studied extensively by Benjamin List, who shared the 2021 Nobel Prize

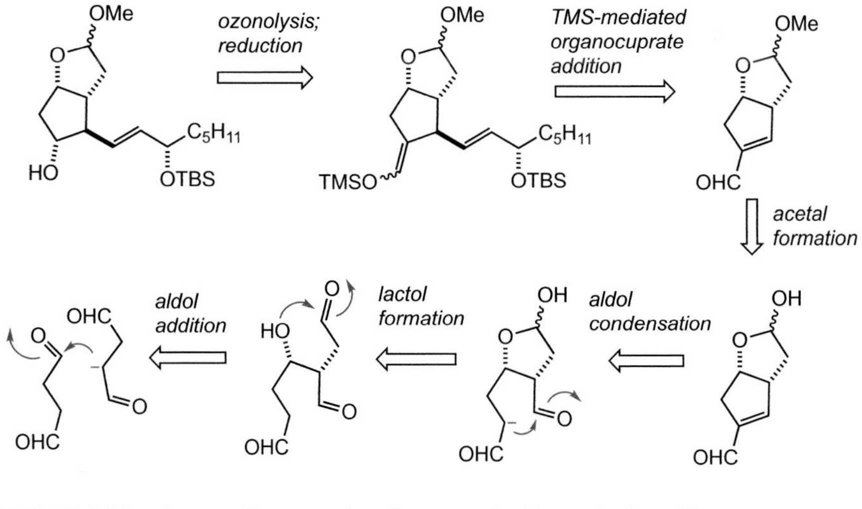

FIGURE 4.10. Aggarwal's approach to the prostaglandin synthesis problem.

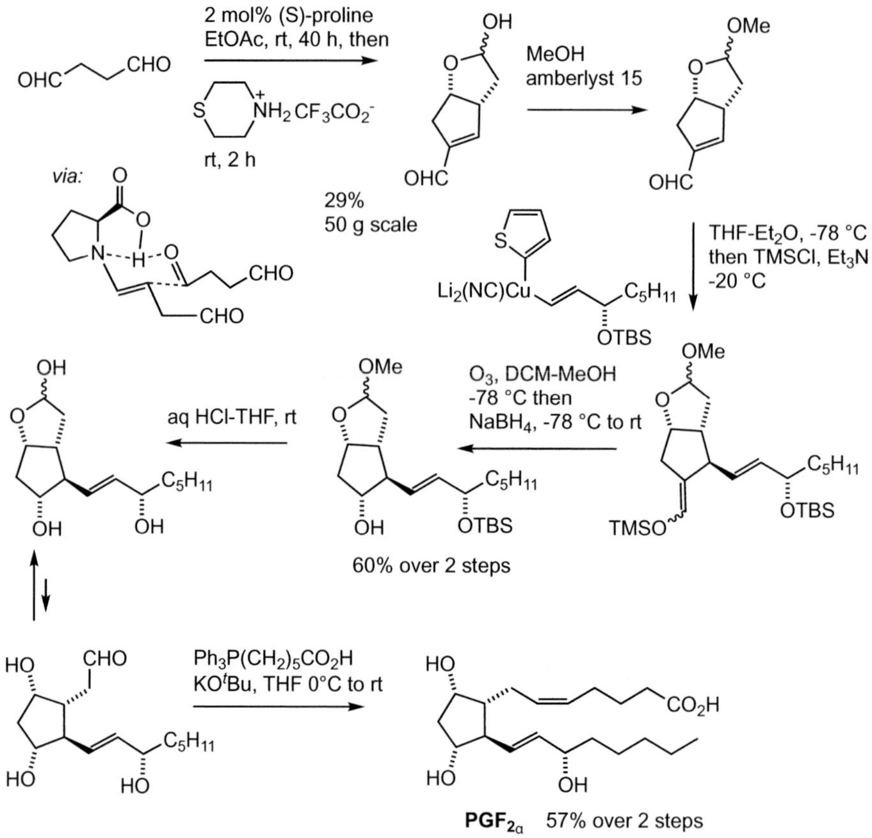

FIGURE 4.11.   Aggarwal's synthesis of PGF$_{2\alpha}$.

in Chemistry for his work in this area. This deceptively simple reaction required extensive optimization to shut down competing pathways and achieve an acceptable level
of chemoselectivity. Thus, it was found that proline was the optimal catalyst for the
first reaction but a poor catalyst for the second. Similarly, dibenzylammonium trifluoroacetate was optimal for the second reaction but a poor catalyst for the first. Further
optimization of the second step led to the use of thiomorpholinium trifluoroacetate as
the catalyst and a reaction temperature of 60 °C. These modifications led to a doubling
of the yield. With such simple, inexpensive starting materials and reagents, the reaction
was readily scaled-up.

The enantiomerically pure enal was subjected to the conjugate addition of a higher
order mixed organocuprate that transfers the intact prostaglandin lower sidechain to
the enal in preference to the thiophene.[8] The enolate intermediate was trapped as a
silyl enol ether. The more electron-rich double bond was selectively ozonized to give
a ketone that was reduced with sodium borohydride to give the target's R-configured
C11 alcohol. The two protecting groups (mixed acetal and TBS ether) were removed,
and the upper prostaglandin sidechain was introduced using Wittig chemistry that

we have already described. Being only seven steps in length and with an ideality of 83%, Aggarwal's versatile enantioselective synthesis of PGF$_{2\alpha}$ is "as good as it gets" when it comes to planning and efficiency.

Most of the reactions that we have used involve heterolytic reorganizations of valence electron pairs as is evident from our arrow-pushing mechanistic rationalizations. The 1980s saw an increased interest in radical reactions, which involve homolytic bond breaking and formation via the movement of single electrons, and the application of free radicals to organic synthesis. The orthogonal-controlled reactivity of organic free radicals as opposed to anionic and cationic species provides good opportunities for the chemoselective manipulation of molecules bearing multiple functional groups. Thus, carbonyls, alcohols, and amines need not be protected during C–C bond-forming reactions of free radicals. Another feature of free radicals is their small steric profile when compared with carbanionic species that usually have metals as well as their ligands associated with them. This property gives free radicals an advantage when making sterically hindered quaternary C–C bonds.

A seminal application of radical chemistry to prostaglandin synthesis came from Gilbert Stork's lab.[9] His synthesis of PGF$_{2\alpha}$ (Figure 4.12) started out with the enzymatic desymmetrization of (1R,3S)-cyclopent-4-ene-1,3-diyl diacetate. This mirrored Noyori's PGF$_{2\alpha}$ opening game but, instead of oxidizing the cyclopentenol

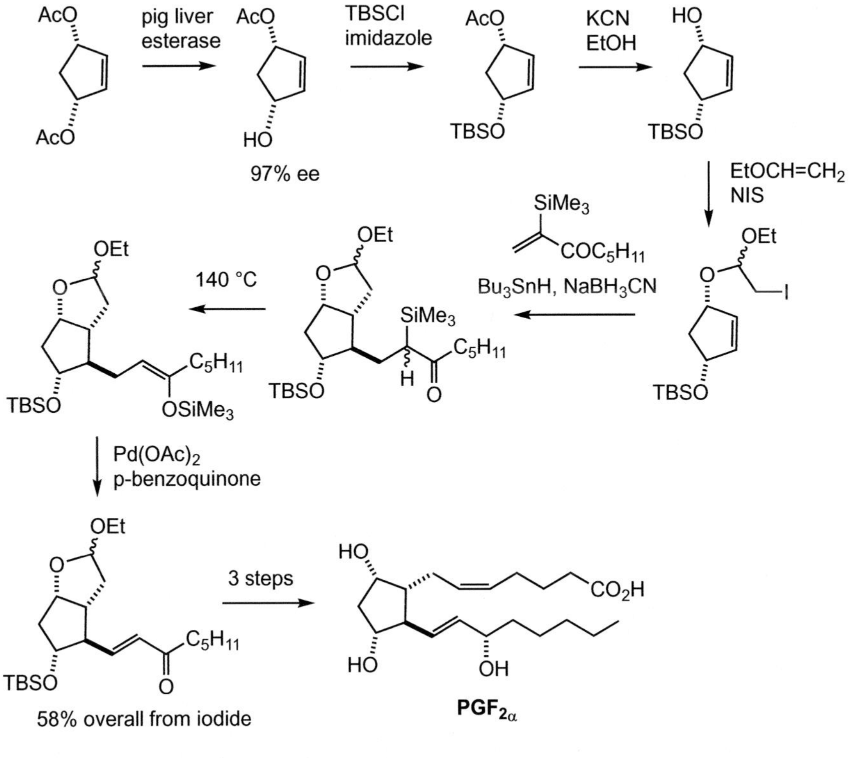

FIGURE 4.12. Stork's radical approach to PGF$_{2\alpha}$.

to a cyclopentanone (see Figure 4.9), he treated it with ethyl vinyl ketone and N-iodosuccinimide (NIS) in ethanol to produce a mixture of iodoether acetal diastereomers. This reaction is related to the previously described iodolactonization in that it also proceeds via an iodonium ion. Photolysis of the iodide in the presence of an α-silylated enone and a low concentration of tributyltin hydride (a good hydrogen atom donor that was generated *in situ* by the reaction of Bu_3SnCl and $NaBH_3CN$) resulted in a radical cascade that had the initially formed radical undergoing a rapid intramolecular 5-exo-trig ring closure (Baldwin's terminology) followed by radical addition to the enone to produce an α-trimethylsilyl ketone. Upon heating, this compound underwent a Brook rearrangement to give a silyl enol ether. This rearrangement involves the [1,3]-migration of a silyl group from the α-carbon to carbonyl oxygen that is driven by favorable thermodynamics (Si–O bonds have a greater bond dissociation energy than Si–C bonds). Exposure of this compound to palladium acetate initiated a Saegusa reaction that resulted in the production of an enone in 58% overall yield. The mechanism of this useful reaction is shown below using the trimethylsilyl enol ether of cyclohexanone as the substrate. In this reaction, Pd (II) forms an oxa-π-allylpalladium complex which undergoes β-hydride elimination to give the enone. The silicon atom played an important role in this reaction by directing the placement of the alkene. The resulting bicyclic acetal could be converted to $PGF_{2\alpha}$ following already established chemistry.

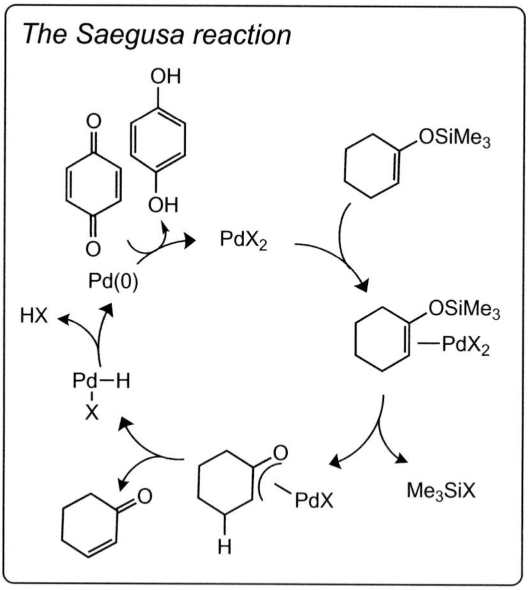

The Saegusa reaction

Stork's and Keck's radical chains:

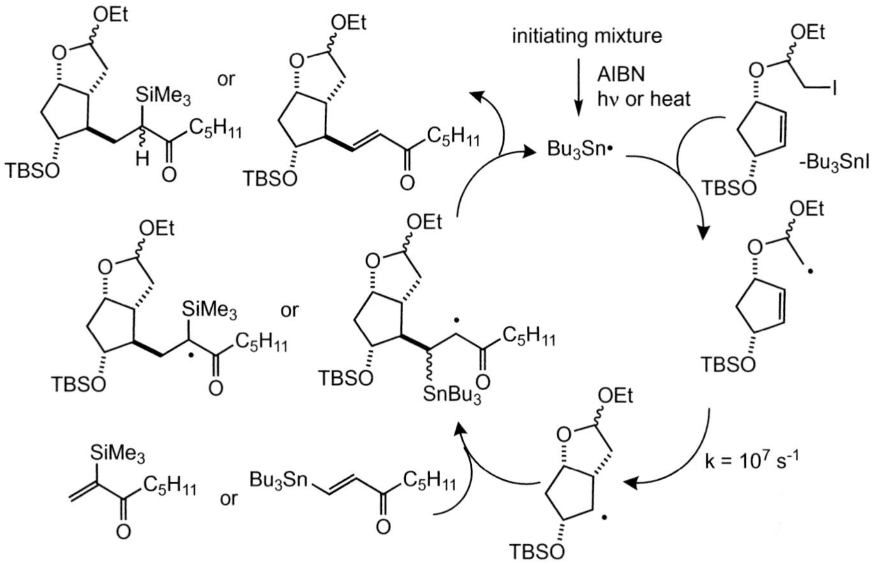

FIGURE 4.13. A head-to-head comparison of Stork's tributyltin hydride radical chain and Keck's simplification of the radical chain through addition to a β -stannyl enone followed by fragmentation to generate Bu$_3$Sn•.

The role of tributyltin hydride in this reaction is to propagate the radical chain by having the terminal radical abstract a hydrogen atom from the tin hydride, generating the tributyltin radical. However, because of its propensity to quench intermediate radicals and terminate the chain reaction prematurely (both are bimolecular processes), the tin hydride was generated *in situ*, thus keeping its concentration low. This would favor unimolecular ring closure and disfavor the early bimolecular radical quenching reaction. An alternative that circumvented the premature quenching problem altogether was desirable. This led Gary Keck to use a β-stannylenone as the radical trap, as it would generate the same product without the need for tin hydride.[10] In this case, the radical intermediate formed by the addition of a radical to the β-stannylenone undergoes an elimination reaction, releasing Bu$_3$Sn• which carries the radical chain. The radical chain for both reactions is shown in Figure 4.13.

The prostaglandin family of natural products has inspired synthetic chemists for more than 70 years not only providing access to the natural structures but also to unnatural synthetic drugs—four examples of which are shown in Figure 4.14.

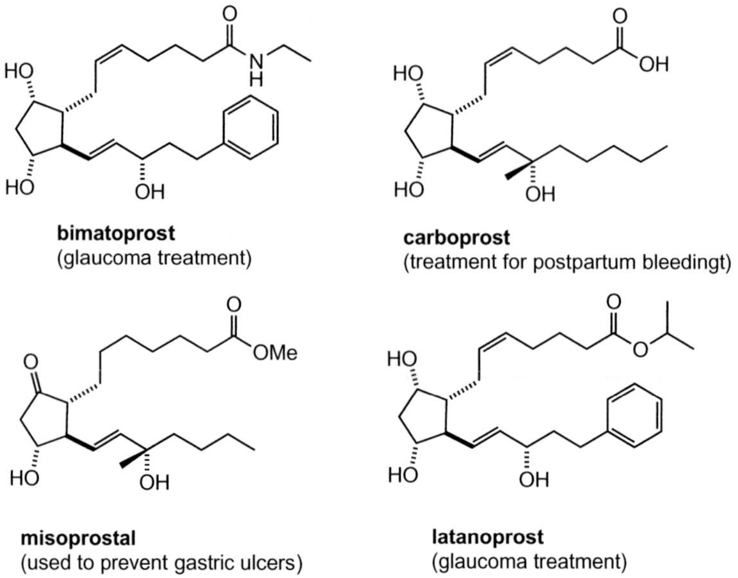

bimatoprost
(glaucoma treatment)

carboprost
(treatment for postpartum bleedingt)

misoprostal
(used to prevent gastric ulcers)

latanoprost
(glaucoma treatment)

FIGURE 4.14. Synthetic drugs that are based on prostaglandins.

TRIQUINANE SYNTHESIS

The prostaglandins are characterized by the presence of a substituted five-membered carbocyclic ring. Hence, the synthetic approaches to these targets have focused on the construction of cyclopentane rings. We will now consider some strategies that have been applied to the triquinane family of sesquiterpenoids, a class of natural products which contain three five-membered carbocyclic rings embedded in rigid compact polycyclic structures. The discussion will begin with Pirrung's synthesis of the angular triquinane isocomene, then we will cover Curran's radical cascade-based synthesis of the linear triquinane hirsutene, and end with Oppolzer and Rawal's approaches to the propellane triquinane modhephene. The molecular structures of these targets are shown in Figure 4.15. Each of them presents unique challenges with respect to their synthesis and provide opportunities to introduce the reader to some powerful transforms for the construction of fused five-membered carbocycles that can be added to your reaction toolbox.

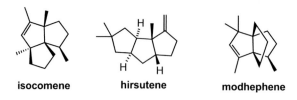

isocomene   **hirsutene**   **modhephene**

FIGURE 4.15. Molecular structures of the three prototype triquinane natural products.

SYNTHESIS OF ISOCOMENE

The prototype angular triquinane, isocomene, was isolated from the rayless golden-rod (*Isocoma wrightii*), a toxic plant that is responsible for livestock poisoning in the southwestern United States and northern Mexico. Pirrung's synthesis of this sesqui-terpene is depicted in Figure 4.16 from superimposed retrosynthetic and synthetic perspectives.[11] Our retrosynthetic analysis of this molecule begins with protonation of the exocyclic olefin to give a tertiary carbenium ion. Application of a reversible Wagner–Meerwein rearrangement converts the [3.3.0] bicyclooctane substructure to a [3.2.1] bicyclooctane. A second Wagner–Meerwein shift leads to a [4.2.0] bicyclooc-tane that, after applying a Wittig transform, reveals the retron for an intramolecular photochemical [2 + 2] cycloaddition reaction. This stereospecific pericyclic reaction provides a reliable method for the synthesis of cyclobutanes. The reversible rear-rangement manifold in the forward direction benefits energetically from the relief of cyclobutane ring strain in going from a [4.2.0] to [3.2.1] system while the driving force for the [3.2.1] to [3.3.0] rearrangement is the formation of a trisubstituted olefin in the final product. Thus, Pirrung's approach benefitted from mechanistic considerations as well as retrosynthetic and synthetic thinking. It should be noted that the direct rear-rangement from the [4.2.0] to the [3.3.0] system by migration of the bridging bond is not stereoelectronically viable because of poor orbital overlap. This less-than-optimal geometry can be visualized three-dimensionally using handheld models.

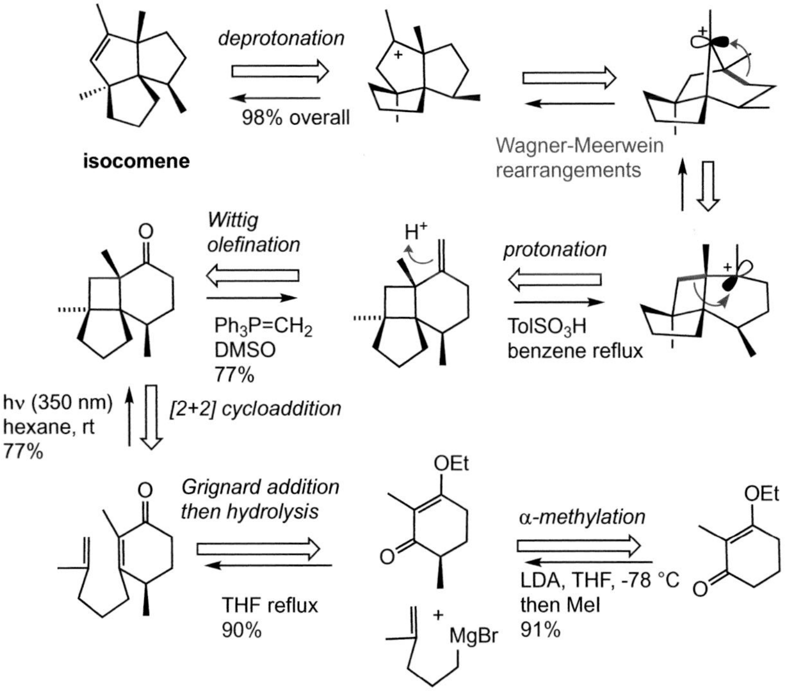

FIGURE 4.16. Pirrung's synthesis of isocomene. The key [4.2.0] to [3.3.0] skeletal rear-rangement via the [3.2.1] intermediate is shown in magenta.

As is often the case with total synthesis projects, the simple scheme showing the successful sequence of reactions belies the difficulties that were encountered along the way. The original plan for converting the tricyclic ketone to the exocyclic olefin involved the addition of a methyl nucleophile such as MeLi to the carbonyl followed by acid-catalyzed dehydration. However, because the Bürgi–Dunitz trajectory (the lowest energy path that a nucleophile takes as it attacks a carbonyl while maintaining maximum orbital overlap between the nucleophile HOMO and the electrophile LUMO)[12] is hindered on both the convex and concave face of the ketone (this can also be seen with a handheld model), conditions could not be found that resulted in nucleophilic addition. Instead, irreversible enolate formation was observed. One might expect the Wittig reaction to have similar problems. However, the Wittig reaction in dimethylsulfoxide (DMSO) succeeded because the enolate can be protonated by DMSO (pKa ~35), generating a small concentration of the dimsyl anion (CH_3SOCH_2:-) reversibly. The ketone can then be siphoned off to the stable Wittig product via le Chartelier's principle. With an ideality of 80%, Pirrung's five-step synthesis of racemic isocomene set a high bar in terms of efficiency and nicely illustrates the value of connecting a specific reaction—in this case sequential Wagner–Meerwein rearrangement—to a specific target. On the downside, this synthesis produced racemic isocomene.

The photochemical (2 + 2) cycloaddition is a powerful reaction that, in this intramolecular example, leads to the formation of cyclobutane ring and, through the tether connecting the olefinic partners, a five-membered carbocyclic ring. Unlike the Diels–Alder cycloaddition that is thermally allowed (enabling the unstrained approach of both the diene and dienophile to each other; see Figure 1.10), the

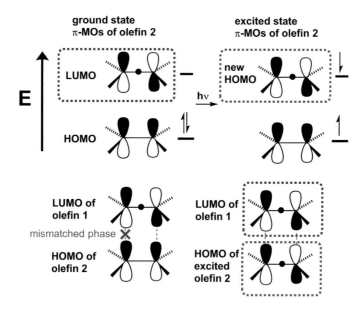

FIGURE 4.17. Qualitative frontier molecular orbital analysis of a [2 + 2] cycloaddition between two alkenes.

suprafacial combination of the HOMO and LUMO of the two reacting olefins in a [2 + 2] cycloaddition is forbidden on orbital symmetry grounds (their phases don't match). This phase problem can be overcome by photochemically exciting an electron from the ground state molecule's HOMO to the LUMO of the excited state as shown in Figure 4.17. Thus, photoexcitation leads to symmetry-matched orbitals and permits the desired [2 + 2] cycloaddition to occur.

SYNTHESIS OF HIRSUTENE

Our next example is Dennis Curran's radical cascade synthesis of the prototype linear triquinane hirsutene, a sesquiterpene natural product isolated from the wood-rotting mushroom *Stereum hirsutum*. Although free radicals were once considered too reactive to be of much use for the synthesis of complex molecules, they are now considered well-behaved enough to be used routinely for the assembly of natural products. Radical-based reactions now form an important set of tools for organic chemists. Free radicals can be extremely selective—a property that renders them useful for natural product synthesis.[13] We saw the usefulness of free radical reactions for the stereocontrolled introduction of acyclic substituents on the core cyclopentane ring of prostaglandins. However, properly designed free-radical cascades can also be used to generate fused five-membered carbocycles as well.

From the synthetic planning perspective, deciding which bonds in a target molecule to break to reveal a radical cascade can be tricky, as the retrons are not so obvious. Often, the best approach involves trying to identify potential starting and ending radicals and then homolytically breaking adjacent C–C bonds and seeing where that leads. The facile formation of five-membered rings generally follows Baldwin's rules for ring closure (which basically state that ring-forming reactions that maintain maximum orbital overlap between the interacting frontier molecular orbitals will be favored). Curran's synthesis of the prototypical linear triquinane hirsutene provides an excellent example of a well-designed radical cascade (Figure 4.18).[14] The key reaction began with the generation of an initiating radical from the thermal decomposition of azobisisobutyronitrile (AIBN). The resulting alkyl radical abstracts an iodide atom from the substrate, forming a primary free radical and stable tributyltin iodide. This alkyl radical is positioned to undergo a rapid 5-exo-trig addition to the cyclopentene, generating a new tertiary alkyl radical that undergoes a 5-exo-dig addition to the acetylene to give the terminal vinyl radical that abstracts a hydrogen atom from the tributyltin hydride to give the final product and regenerate the carrier tributyltin radical.

The first ring closure benefits from a gem-dimethyl effect, which can dramatically increase the rate of cyclizations.[15] Although the mechanism of this effect is still under debate, one possible explanation is that the gem-dimethyl group *destabilizes* acyclic conformations (rotamers) in which the reactive functionality are too far apart from each other to interact. This increases the effective concentration of rotamers that place the reactive functionality within the range needed for bond formation, leading to reaction rate enhancements.

The preparation of the substrate for the radical cascade is shown in Figure 4.19. Application of Ireland's modification of the Claisen rearrangement to the allylic

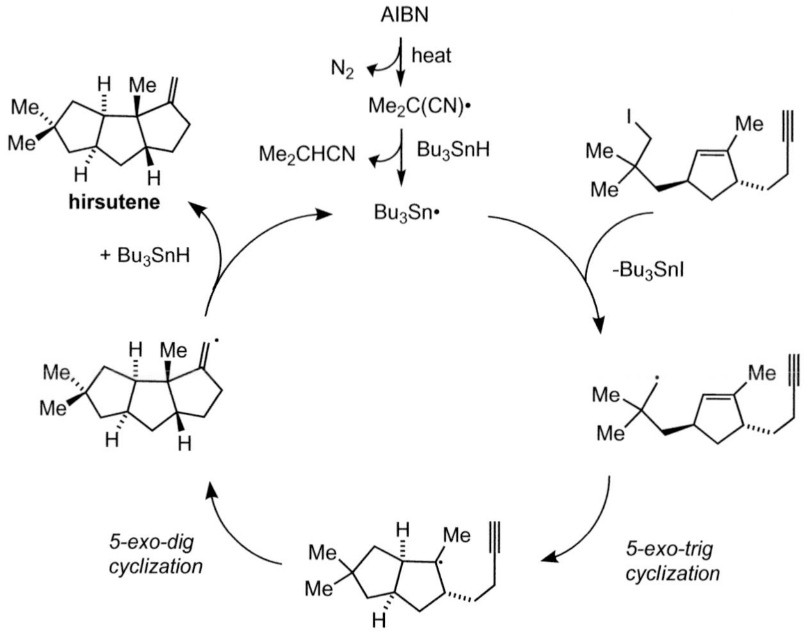

FIGURE 4.18. The key radical cascade in Curran's synthesis of hirsutene.

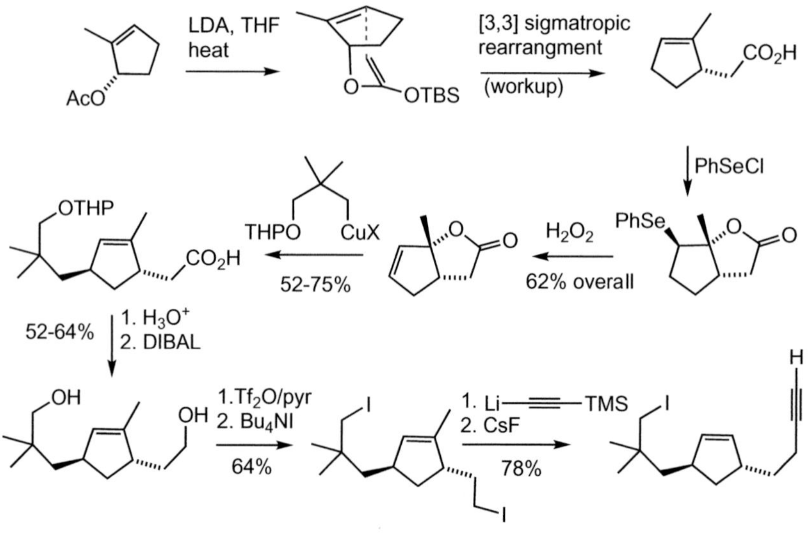

FIGURE 4.19. Synthesis of the substrate for Curran's radical cascade.

acetate (readily available in enantiomerically pure form) produced a γ,δ-unsaturated carboxylic acid after workup.[16] Treatment of this compound with phenylselenyl chloride resulted in anti-addition to the olefin via a three-membered heterocyclic intermediate. This reaction is analogous to halolactonization. Oxidation of the selenide to a selenoxide followed by thermally induced syn-elimination produced an allylic lactone that underwent an S_N2' reaction with an organocuprate to give a trisubstituted cyclopentene. This compound was converted to a diiodide via a bis-triflate that underwent regioselective displacement at the unhindered C–I bond (the less reactive iodide being neopentyl) by a lithium acetylide yielding the substrate for the radical cascade after removal of the TMS (trimethylsilyl) protecting group. Application of the radical cascade afforded racemic hirsutene in 53% yield. This 11-step synthesis of hirsutene had a respectable ideality of 45%.

SYNTHESIS OF MODHEPHENE

Modhephene is the prototypical propellane triquinane. Along with the angular triquinane isocomene, it is also isolated from the rayless goldenrod. An efficient eight-step synthesis of racemic modhephene was reported by Oppolzer (Figure 4.20).[17] The key retrosynthetic disconnection involved an ene transform/reaction. The synthesis began with Darzens–Kondakov acylation of cyclopentene with 3,3-dimethylacryloyl chloride. Upon heating, the 1,4-pentadien-3-one moiety underwent a Nazarov electrocyclization to give a bicyclo [3.3.0] system that contained

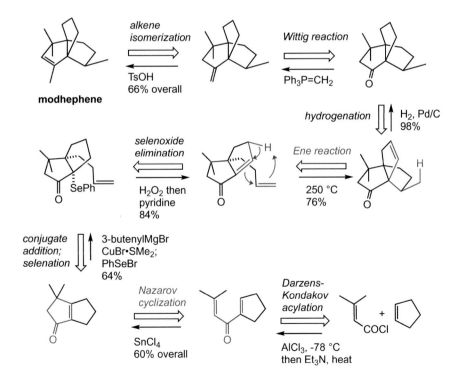

FIGURE 4.20. Oppolzer's "ene approach" to modhephene. The key transforms/reactions are colored magenta.

an enone moiety. The conjugate addition of a butenyl cuprate produced an enolate that was trapped with phenylselenyl bromide to give the α-selenide. Oxidation with hydrogen peroxide produced a selenoxide that underwent spontaneous elimination to the dienone. This compound was set up for the key ene reaction. This concerted pericyclic reaction proceeded at 250 °C and generated the third cyclopentane ring and installed the secondary methyl group stereospecifically. Note that modhephene does not contain the complete retron for the indicated ene reaction, so a double bond had to be installed to enable application of the ene transform. The final steps in the synthesis involved hydrogenation of the alkene, Wittig olefination, and the thermodynamically driven isomerization of the resulting exocyclic olefin to its trisubstituted endocyclic isomer. This eight-step synthesis afforded racemic modhephene in 16% overall yield with a 50% ideality.

The key strategic reactions in this synthesis were the Nazarov cyclization and the ene reaction. These pericyclic reactions may not be familiar, so their mechanisms will be briefly discussed (Figure 4.21). The Nazarov cyclization is a concerted electrocyclic reaction whose orbital symmetry implications can be understood by looking at the HOMO of a pentadienyl cation. Formation of a five-membered ring results from a conrotatory motion of the terminal sp^2 carbons. The ene reaction is analogous to a sigmatropic rearrangement. Thus, the easiest way to see the orbital symmetry requirements is to break the migrating C–H bond homolytically. Once done, there

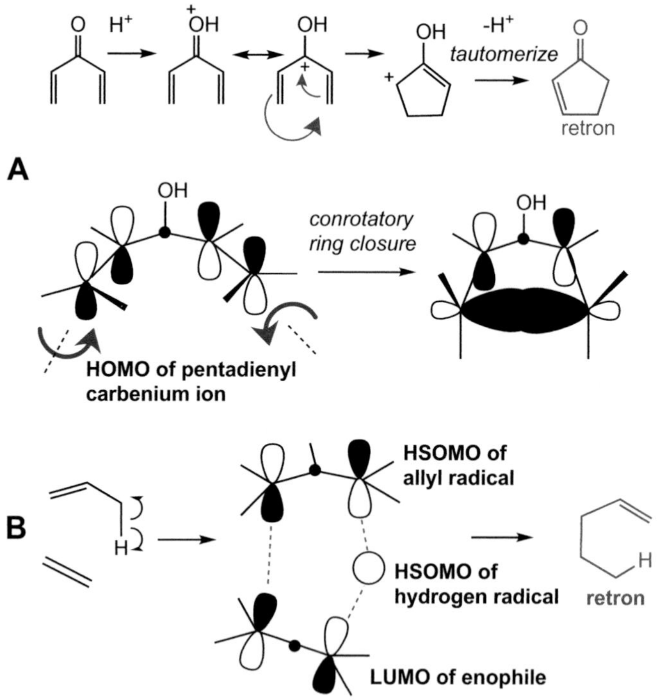

FIGURE 4.21.   Frontier molecular orbital analysis of (A) the Nazarov cyclization and (B) the ene reaction.

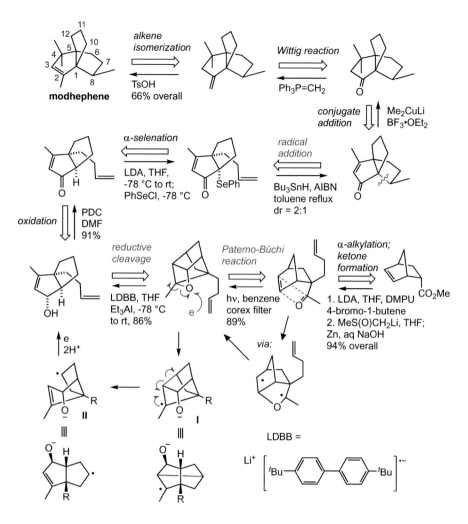

FIGURE 4.22. Rawal's radical approach to modhephene.

is an allyl radical and a hydrogen radical. The least strained combination of the ene component HOMOs and the LUMO of the enophile component can be seen to involve suprafacial interactions.

Among the chemical approaches to modhephene that have been reported over the years, the synthesis by Rawal[18] stands out in terms of its innovation and potential for enantioselectivity (Figure 4.22). Working retrosynthetically, the first key bond disconnection is at C1–C8, the same disconnection that was seen in Oppolzer's mod-hephene synthesis. However, in this case, the bond is formed by a 5-exo-trig radi-cal addition to the pendant alkene. This disconnection makes good sense in accord with Corey's topological rules: it involves a five-membered ring, occurs at a bridge, and eliminates a stereocenter. The molecule that results from the radical addition is actually one that Oppolzer made during his modhephene synthesis, so reaching this point would constitute a formal synthesis of the target. The next key structure was a substituted bicyclo[3.3.0]octane system that resulted from the serial application of three powerful transforms, (1) reductive cleavage of a caged oxetane, (2) an intramolecular Paternò–Büchi reaction, and (3) a Diels–Alder reaction to construct the acetylnorbornene Paternò–Büchi substrate.

The Paternò–Büchi cycloaddition, like the dimerization of ethylene, requires photolytic excitation. However, unlike the concerted cycloadditions that we have seen thus far, a mixture of mechanisms involving radical intermediates may be at play. The bond reorganization begins with the promotion of an electron from a carbonyl nonbonding orbital to an antibonding orbital (n to π^* transition) and proceeds through a diradical intermediate. The intramolecular caged oxetane is produced in good yield. Because of its inherent angle strain, the oxetane C–O bonds are susceptible to reductive cleavage by lithium di-t-butyl-biphenylide. Mechanistically, this is accomplished by the addition of electrons to the σ^* antibonding orbital, producing a radical anion upon cleavage (Structure **I**). The observed regioselectivity (which C–O bond of the oxetane is broken) favors formation of the tertiary radical. A second strain-driven cleavage occurs to give the final radical anion (Structure **II**) that picks up a second electron to give a dianion that is protonated upon workup. The resulting allylic alcohol is then carried forward to the propellane as shown.

Rawal's 10-step synthesis of the propellane triquinane modhephene proceeded in 43% overall yield starting from a readily available Diels–Alder cycloadduct and had an 80% ideality, underscoring its efficiency. This group also showed that the Paternò–Büchi based strategy could be extended to the angular and linear triquinanes as well, highlighting the generality of this approach.

SUMMARY

Collectively, the approaches to prostaglandin and triquinane synthesis covered in this chapter provide excellent illustrations of holistic synthetic planning. Starting with E. J. Corey's classical approach to prostaglandin $PGF_{2\alpha}$, we saw how total synthesis can serve as a catalyst for the development of new synthetic methods. This was followed by a survey of some alternative approaches to prostaglandins that included conjugate addition/enolate trapping, a very practical organocatalytic synthesis, and the use of radical cascades. We then turned our attention to the synthesis of triquinanes, focusing on efficient syntheses isocomene, hirsutene, and modhephene. The syntheses integrate retrospective and prospective thinking, an appreciation of molecular structure and reactivity, and the use of multiple strategies and tactics. A variety of reactions were introduced, focusing on the construction of fused cyclopentane rings.

TUTORIAL: PLANNING A SYNTHESIS OF SEYCHELLENE

In this tutorial, you will get more practice performing retrosynthetic analysis using the sesquiterpenoid seychellene as our synthetic target. This small (MW 204) compact molecule contains four fused cyclohexane rings and five stereocenters. We start our analysis by applying topological strategies to disassemble the polycyclic ring system and then add functionality to enable both Diels–Alder and radical addition transforms. We will then assess the viability of the resulting branches of the hypothetical synthesis tree based on relevant mechanistic considerations.

seychellene

Step 1: Identify functional groups in the target molecule noting if they activate proximal carbon atoms. There is only one functional group in the target molecule: the exo-methylene group located on one of the 2-carbon bridges.

Step 2: Identify patterns that may suggest simplifying disconnections or the use of powerful transforms. If necessary, add functional groups to create powerful retrons. Employing a topological strategy, we can see that cleavage of each of the four bridging bonds in the bicyclo[2.2.2] ring result in substituted decalin systems. Disconnection **D** looks especially promising because, with minimal alteration, it can accommodate α-alkylation and Diels–Alder transforms. Disconnection **A** produces a structure that has an extra stereocenter compared to **B**, **C**, and **D**; disconnection **B** contains a difficult-to-make quaternary carbon; and disconnection **C** would require more extensive alteration. Thus, these three disconnections are given a lower priority.

seychellene

With **D**, a pattern begins to emerge that suggests straightforward modifications that will produce a powerful intermolecular Diels–Alder retron. However, the retron is obscured to a certain extent because it consists of a labile combination of silyl enol ether and a β-methoxy group, which spontaneously decomposes to the cyclohexanone upon acidic aqueous workup. Thus, it is better to think of the cyclohexanone substructure as the retron for a Diels–Alder reaction of a 1-methoxy-3-siloxy diene. Siloxy dienes are descendants of the parent (E)-1-methoxy-3-trimethysilyl-1,3-butadiene, which is known as the Danishefsky–Kitahara diene (often simply referred to as the Danishefsky diene). The result of such substitution is a diene that is more reactive (higher HOMO energy resulting in a smaller HOMO–LUMO gap) and that possesses more asymmetrical orbital coefficients (leading to increased regioselectivity with unsymmetrical dienophiles) as well as potential activation of all four diene carbons.[19]

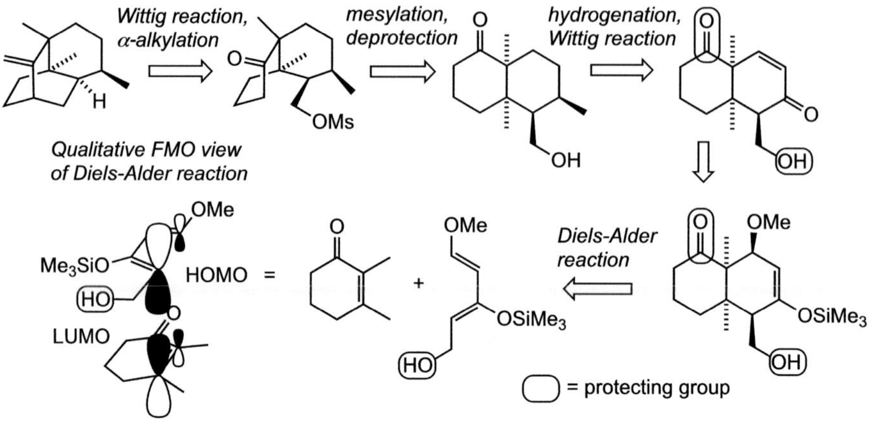

Qualitative FMO view of Diels-Alder reaction

◯ = protecting group

Sometimes it pays to disregard the rules or, at least, bend them. Such is the case if we cleave a bond that leads to a bridged rather than a fused ring system as shown below.

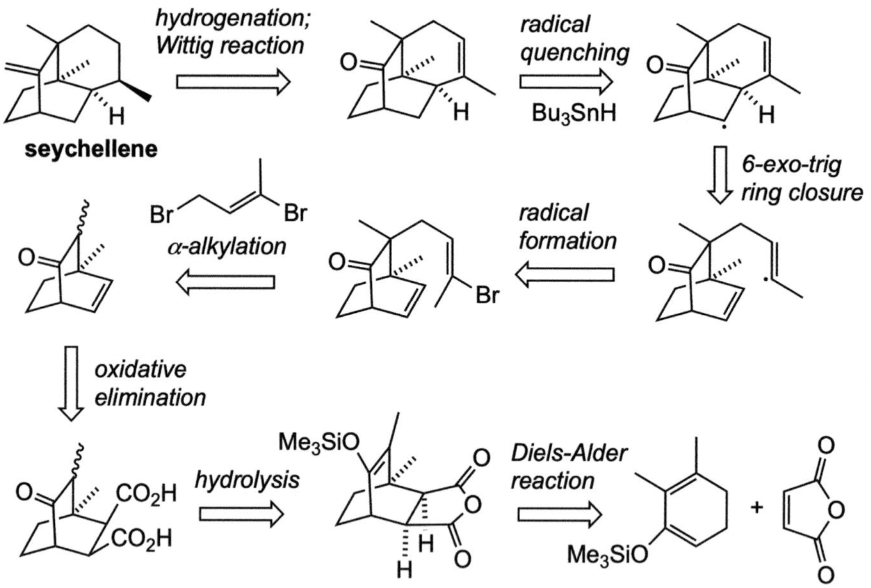

The sequence begins with the application of Wittig and hydrogenation transforms, leading to a structure that contains a radical addition retron. The vinyl radical formed by abstraction of a bromine atom adds to the alkene via a 6-exo-trig transition state that adheres to Baldwin's rules for closure, foregoing the possible 5-exo-trig addition to the ketone for the free radical chemoselectivity reasons that we mentioned earlier. The 3-bromo-2-butenyl moiety can be installed by alkylating the ketone enolate on its less hindered face. The bicyclo[2.2.2]octane ring system contains a hidden Diels–Alder retron that requires a decarboxylative oxidative elimination (using lead tetraacetate) to reveal the cyclohexene. For the Diels–Alder reaction, a hydrolysis transform leads to a silyl enol ether and anhydride that actuate a Diels–Alder reaction between a siloxy activated diene and a highly electron-deficient symmetric maleic anhydride dienophile. This route was used by Stork in his synthesis of seychellene.[20] A simpler Diels–Alder reaction between a ketene equivalent and 1-methylcyclohexa-1,3-diene can also be proposed but would be rejected on the grounds that the diene substitution would favor the wrong regioisomer on FMO grounds. In the retrosynthetic analysis we just performed, we restricted ourselves to making a single initial bond disconnection that was guided by the target's topology, according to the rules developed by Corey. These disconnections resulted in simpler structures. We then shifted to a transform-based strategy, looking for or creating retrons that are associated with specific reactions.

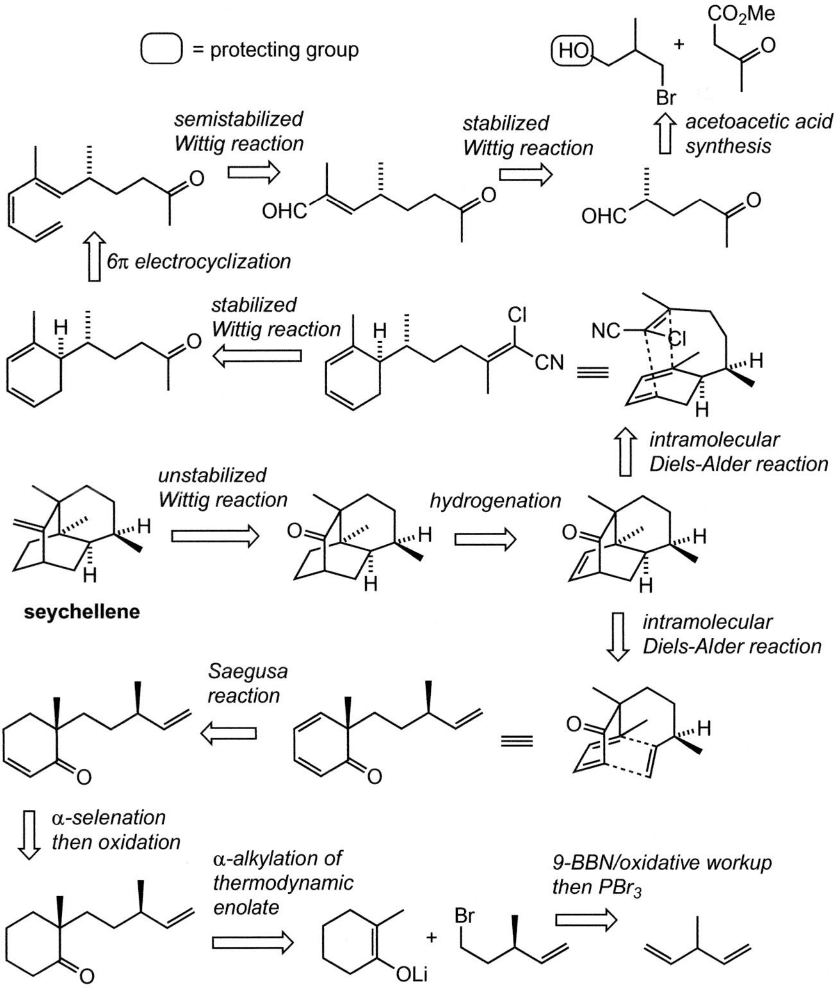

We can also start out with a transform-based strategy, looking for or creating powerful Diels–Alder retrons in the target molecule. Thus, by adding a double bond to the unsubstituted ethylene bridge, we enable two intramolecular Diels–Alder transforms. One of these intramolecular Diels–Alder reactions has a ketene equivalent reacting with a tethered cyclohexadiene to form the bicyclo[2.2.2]octane system while the other possibility involves a cyclohexadienone reacting with a tethered unactivated alkene. The latter is an example of an inverse electron demand Diels–Alder reaction in which the FMO interactions are between an electron-deficient diene LUMO and the dienophile HOMO. Note that the cycloexadienone is prevented from tautomerizing to an aromatic phenol by the intervention of a quaternary carbon in the ring. This disconnection was actually employed by Yoshikoshi in his synthesis of seychellene.[21]

REFERENCES

1. Corey, E. J., Schaaf, T. K., Huber, W., Koelliker, U., & Weinshenker, N. M. (1970). Total synthesis of prostaglandins $F_2\alpha$ and E_2 as the naturally occuring forms. *Journal of the American Chemical Society*, *92*(2), 397–398.
2. Shiner, C. S., Fisher, A. M., & Yacoby, F. (1983). Intermediacy of α-chloro amides in the basic hydrolysis of α-chloro nitriles to ketones. *Tetrahedron Letters*, *24*(51), 5687–5690.
3. Corey, E. J., & Loh, T. P. (1991). First application of attractive intramolecular interactions to the design of chiral catalysts for highly enantioselective Diels-Alder reactions. *Journal of the American Chemical Society*, *113*(23), 8966–8967.
4. Corey, E. J., Bakshi, R. K., Shibata, S., Chen, C. P., & Singh, V. K. (1987). A stable and easily prepared catalyst for the enantioselective reduction of ketones. Applications to multistep syntheses. *Journal of the American Chemical Society*, *109*(25), 7925–7926.
5. Corey, E. J., & Venkateswarlu, A. (1972). Protection of hydroxyl groups as tert-butyldimethylsilyl derivatives. *Journal of the American Chemical Society*, *94*(17), 6190–6191.
6. Noyori, R., & Suzuki, M. (1993). Organic synthesis of prostaglandins: Advancing biology. *Science*, *259*(5091), 44–45.
7. (a) Coulthard, G., Erb, W., & Aggarwal, V. K. (2012). Stereocontrolled organocatalytic synthesis of prostaglandin $PGF_2\alpha$ in seven steps. *Nature*, *489*(7415), 278–281. (b) Bennett, S. H., Coulthard, G., & Aggarwal, V. K. (2020). Prostaglandin total synthesis enabled by the organocatalytic dimerization of succinaldehyde. *The Chemical Record*, *20*(9), 936–947.
8. Lipshutz, B. H., Kozlowski, J. A., Parker, D. A., Nguyen, S. L., & McCarthy, K. E. (1985). More highly mixed, higher order cyanocuprates "R_T(2-thienyl) Cu(CN)Li$_2$". Efficient reagents which promote selective ligand transfer. *Journal of Organometallic Chemistry*, *285*(1–3), 437–447.
9. Stork, G., Sher, P. M., & Chen, H. L. (1986). Radical cyclization-trapping in the synthesis of natural products. A simple, stereocontrolled route to prostaglandin $F_2\alpha$. *Journal of the American Chemical Society*, *108*(20), 6384–6385.
10. Keck, G. E., & Burnett, D. A. (1987). β.-Stannyl enones as radical traps: A very direct route to $PGF_2\alpha$. *The Journal of Organic Chemistry*, *52*(13), 2958–2960.
11. Pirrung, M. C. (1981). Total synthesis of (+)-isocomene and related studies. *Journal of the American Chemical Society*, *103*(1), 82–87.
12. Bürgi, H. B., Dunitz, J. D., Lehn, J. M., & Wipff, G. (1974). Stereochemistry of reaction paths at carbonyl centres. *Tetrahedron*, *30*(12), 1563–1572.

13. Jasperse, C. P., Curran, D. P., & Fevig, T. L. (1991). Radical reactions in natural product synthesis. *Chemical Reviews*, *91*(6), 1237–1286.

14. Curran, D. P., & Rakiewicz, D. M. (1985). Tandem radical approach to linear condensed cyclopentanoids. Total synthesis of (+)-Hirsutene. *Journal of the American Chemical Society*, *107*(5), 1448–1449.

15. Jung, M. E., & Piizzi, G. (2005). gem-Disubstituent effect: Theoretical basis and synthetic applications. *Chemical Reviews*, *105*(5), 1735–1766.

16. Ireland, R. E., & Mueller, R. H. (1972). Claisen rearrangement of allyl esters. *Journal of the American Chemical Society*, *94*(16), 5897–5898.

17. Oppolzer, W., & Bättig, K. (1981). A short and efficient synthesis of (±)-modhephene by a stereoelectronically-controlled ene-reaction. *Helvetica Chimica Acta*, *64*(7), 2489–2491.

18. Dvorak, C. A., & Rawal, V. H. (1997). Synthesis of the naturally occurring [3.3.3] propellane (±)-modhephene featuring a photocycloaddition–reductive fragmentation diquinane construction. *Chemical Communications*, *24*(24), 2381–2382.

19. Danishefsky, S. (1981). Siloxy dienes in total synthesis. *Accounts of Chemical Research*, *14*(12), 400–406.

20. Stork, G., & Baine, N. H. (1985). Vinyl radical cyclization in the synthesis of natural products: Seychellene. *Tetrahedron Letters*, *26*(48), 5927–5930.

21. Fukamiya, N., Kato, M., & Yoshikoshi, A. (1973). Total synthesis of (±)-seychellene. *Journal of the Chemical Society, Perkin Transactions*, *1*, 1843–1847.

PRACTICE PROBLEMS

1. Calculate the percent ideality of Corey's synthesis of $PGF_{2\alpha}$ and those of Noyori, Aggarwal, and Stork. Which one is the most efficient?

2. Outline a synthesis of the following marine eicosanoid. Include a retrosynthetic analysis and a forward synthetic plan that includes reagents to be used or a description of the desired transformation.

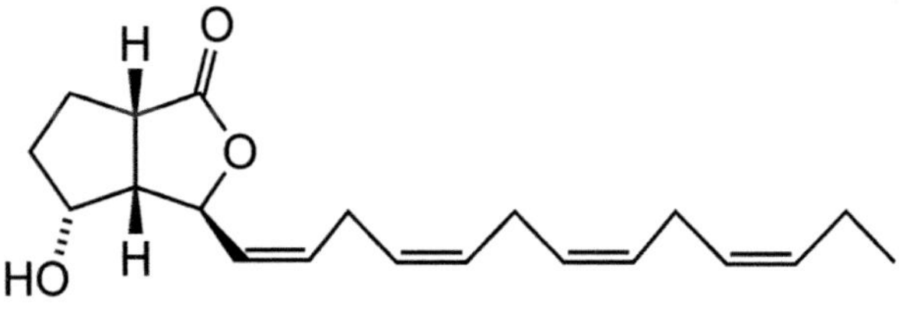

3. Provide an arrow-pushing mechanism for the following reaction.

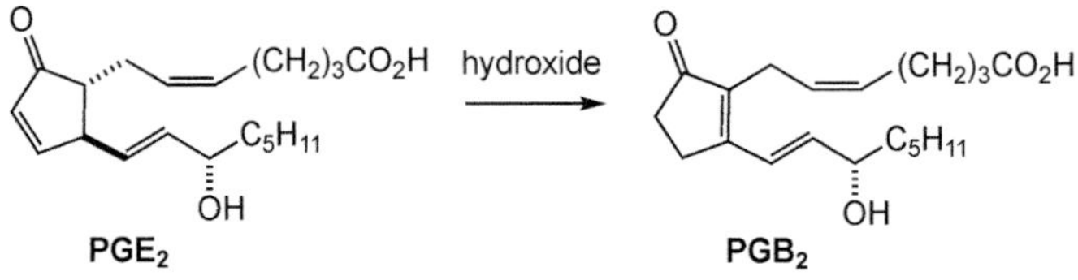

4. What is the product of the following reaction?

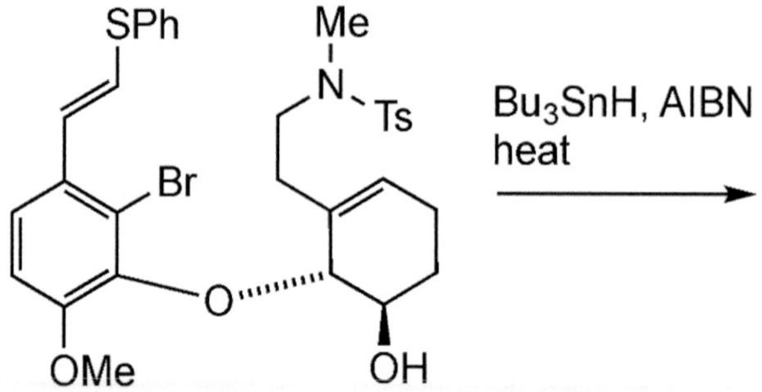

5. The Diels–Alder reaction can be used to introduce acyclic functionality and stereocenters. Show how a Diels–Alder reaction can be used to synthesize the highly functionalized pyrrolidine on the far right.

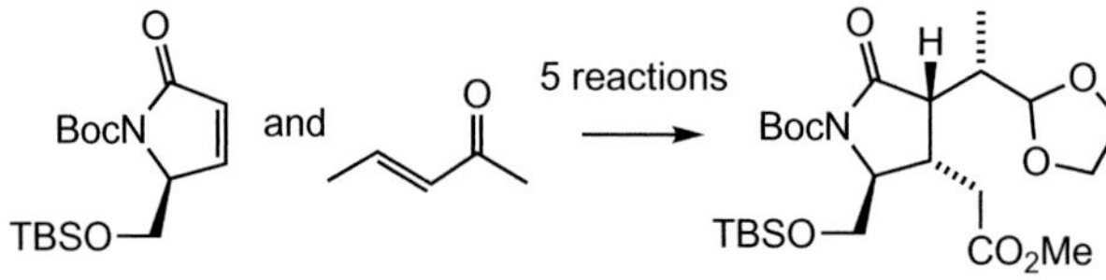

6. Draw out the radical chain for Rawal's radical addition that formed the propellane structure in his modhephene synthesis.

7. Show how you could make Curran's synthesis of hirsutene and Rawal's synthesis of modhephene enantioselective.

8. Critically assess the feasibility of the syntheses proposed for the intramolecular Diels–Alder routes to seychellene in this chapter's tutorial.

5 Polyketide Synthesis
The Challenge of Acyclic Stereocontrol

CONCEPTS AND REACTIONS INTRODUCED IN CHAPTER 5:

- **The B-Alkyl Suzuki cross-coupling reaction** (Miyaura, N., Ishiyama, T., Ishikawa, M., & Suzuki, A. (1986). Palladium-catalyzed cross-coupling reactions of B-alkyl-9-BBN or trialkylboranes with aryl and 1-alkenyl halides. *Tetrahedron letters*, *27*(52), 6369–6372.)
- **Nozaki–Hiyama–Kishi (NHK) allylation reaction** (Hiyama, T., Okude, Y., Kimura, K., & Nozaki, H. (1982). Highly selective carbon-carbon bond forming reactions mediated by chromium (II) reagents. *Bulletin of the Chemical Society of Japan*, *55*(2), 561–568.)
- **Asymmetric aldol addition using chiral enolates** (Evans, D. A., Takacs, J. M., McGee, L. R., Ennis, M. D., Mathre, D. J., & Bartroli, J. (1981). Chiral enolate design. *Pure and Applied Chemistry*, *53*(6), 1109–1127.)
- **Yamaguchi macrolactonization** (Majhi, S. (2021). Applications of Yamaguchi method to esterification and macrolactonization in total synthesis of bioactive natural products. *ChemistrySelect*, *6*(17), 4178–4206.)
- **Hydrozirconation of alkynes** (Schwartz, J., & Labinger, J. A. (1976). Hydrozirconation: a new transition metal reagent for organic synthesis. *Angewandte Chemie International Edition in English*, *15*(6), 333–340.)

POLYKETIDES

Polyketides are a large and varied class of natural products that includes some very important antibiotics. The structures of five polyketides that will be discussed in this chapter are shown in Figure 5.1. These specific molecules were chosen for reasons of historical significance and because they contain multiple stereocenters and functional groups that provide opportunities to develop effective strategies and supporting tactics for synthetic planning. R. B. Woodward recognized the challenge associated with the synthesis of polyketides when he commented[1] on the archetypical macrocyclic polyketide antibiotic, erythromycin: "Erythromycin, with all our advantages, looks at present quite hopelessly complex, particularly in view of its plethora of asymmetric centers." Of course, this opinion was offered nearly seven decades ago. We shall see that organic synthesis has progressed to the point where this pessimistic prediction is no longer true.

Erythromycin is a macrolide antibiotic (a macrolide is a polyketide having eight or more skeletal atoms in its main lactone ring; erythromycin has a 14-membered

DOI: 10.1201/9781003369431-5

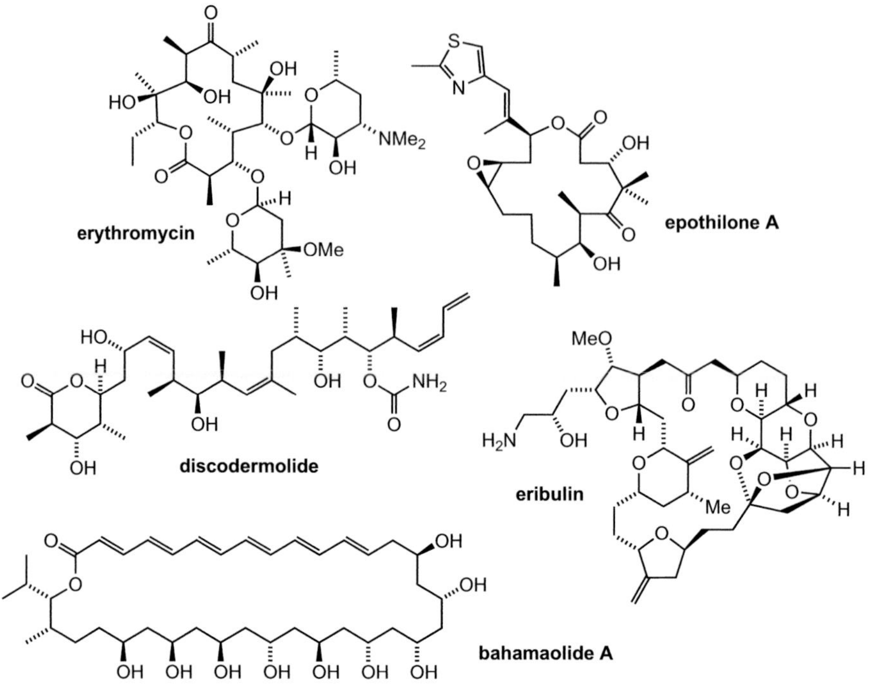

FIGURE 5.1.   Structures of the five polyketide target molecules discussed in this chapter.

lactone) that is used to treat bacterial infections, while the epothilones (which contain a 16-membered lactone) and discodermolide (which contains only a six-membered lactone and is not a macrolide) exhibit anticancer activities that are analogous to that of paclitaxel (they both interrupt mitosis by inhibiting microtubule disassembly). Both erythromycin and epothilone A are isolated from culturable soil bacteria, whereas discodermolide is obtained (with some difficulty) in minute quantities from a deep sea marine sponge (0.002% from frozen material) making total synthesis the most reliable source for biological investigations. Bahamaolide A (a 36-membered lactone), which is isolated from marine sediment, shows activity against pathogenic fungi. Its total synthesis confirmed the structural assignment of this structurally complex natural product. Eribulin is a truncated analogue of the marine natural product halichondrin B, a sponge-derived anticancer agent. It is noteworthy for being the most structurally complex drug produced by chemical synthesis.

The biosynthesis of polyketides is performed by modular polyketide synthetases that are comprised of multiple proteins with proximal functional domains that act as assembly lines for the stepwise construction of these natural products. The synthetase for 6-deoxyerythronolide B, the biosynthetic precursor to the erythromycins, is shown schematically in Figure 5.2. Each module is responsible for a specific transformation as the polyketide skeleton is elongated and processed to give a unique polyketide product. The sequence begins with the attachment of a propionate unit

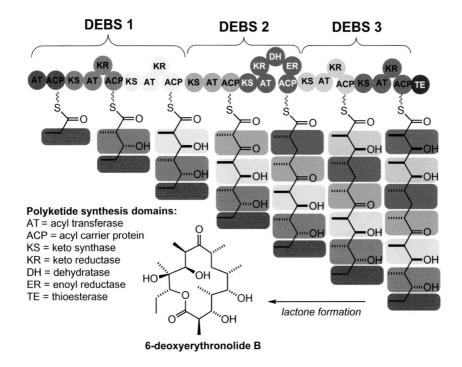

FIGURE 5.2. Modular biosynthesis of 6-deoxyerythronolide B (DEB) by DEB synthetase (DEBS) subunits 1-3.

((HO$_2$C)CH(Me)COSR) to an acyl carrier protein via a decarboxylative Claisen reaction. The resulting β-ketothioester may then be modified by reduction to give an aldol. Dehydration produces an α,β-unsaturated thioester that may be reduced further to introduce a methylene group. In the case of the macrolides, when the linear skeleton is complete, the assembled chain cyclizes by protein-guided hydroxyl attack on the thioester to form a lactone.

ERYTHRONOLIDE B

Let's begin our discussion with the retrosynthetic disconnections in E. J. Corey's synthesis of erythronolide B,[2] which provides an excellent example of synthetic planning (Figure 5.3). Erythronolide B is a biosynthetic precursor of erythromycin A, which has monosaccharides attached to the 3- and 5- positions and a methyl group at C12. The erythromycins are isolated from the bacterium *Saccharopolyspora erythraea*, and their analogues are used around the world as antibiotics. Although erythronolide B contains a 14-membered ring, like other macrolides, it maintains a relatively stable conformation in solution. The three-dimensional (3-D) structure of this molecule is approximated by the first molecule depicted in Figure 5.3. The three-dimensionality of erythronolide B and all macrolides is generally due to the ring substituents' effect

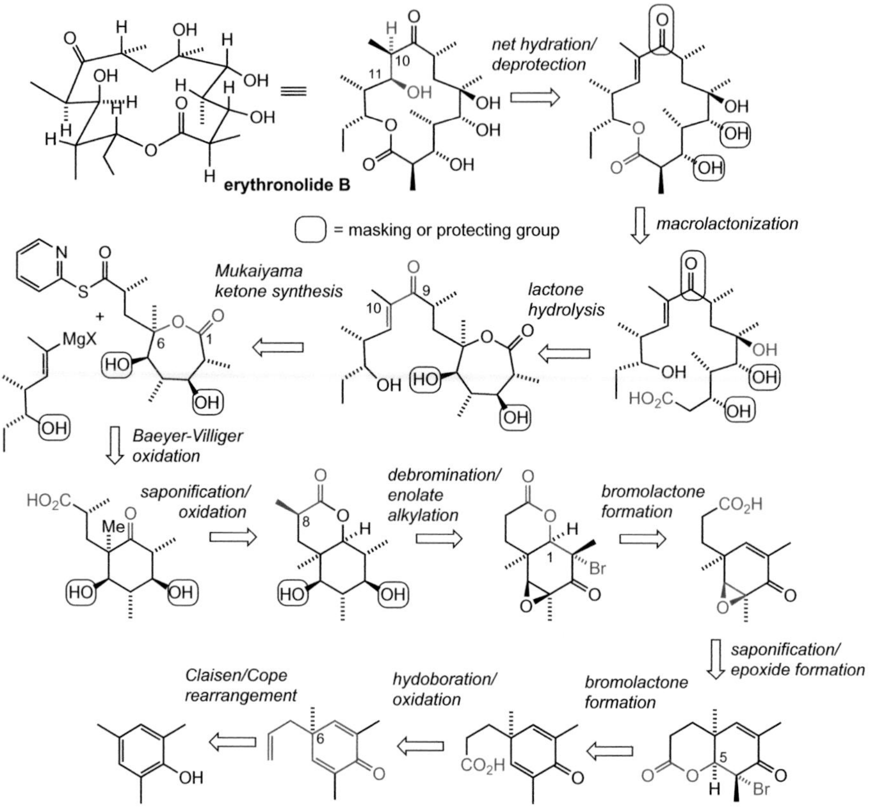

FIGURE 5.3. Retrosynthetic disconnections in Corey's erythronolide B synthesis. (Retrons are colored magenta).

on the macrocyclic conformation and must be kept in mind even if the macrocyclic structures are depicted as "flat." The conformational rigidity associated with such macrocycles can influence their chemical reactivity and biological properties.

The first skeletal bond disconnection involves cleavage of the macrocyclic lactone bond, which leads to a linear hydroxy acid. In a seemingly nonproductive (nonsimplifying) step, a seven-membered lactone is formed by the condensation of the 1-carboxylic acid and 6-hydroxyl group. The logic behind this move will soon become apparent. Meanwhile, the enone is the retron for a mild acylation reaction, developed by the Japanese chemist Teruaki Mukaiyama, that involved the addition of a vinylic Grignard reagent to a 2-pyridine thioester. At low temperatures, the tetrahedral intermediate that results from this addition is stabilized by chelation and does not collapse to a ketone, which would be attacked by unreacted Grignard reagent. However, after decomposing any excess Grignard reagent, the chelate is disrupted, and the ketone is revealed by an aqueous workup. This disconnection divided the molecule approximately in half, greatly simplifying the synthesis problem. Returning to the ketone, the application of a Baeyer–Villiger transform accounts for the formation of a highly functionalized seven-membered caprolactone. The cyclohexanone substrate for the Baeyer–Villiger reaction possesses a hidden C_2-symmetry plane that is revealed in the precursor to sequential bidirectional bromolactonizations. The C_2-symmetric cyclohex-2,5-en-1-one-4-propionic acid was prepared from 2,4,6-trimethylphenol via tandem Claisen/Cope rearrangements and olefin oxidation.

Switching to the forward direction, Corey's synthesis of the C1–C9 segment of erythronolide B (Figure 5.4) began with the C-allylation of 2,4,6-trimethylphenol via sequential Claisen and Cope rearrangements. The vinyl group was then converted to a carboxylic acid with a hydroboration/Jones oxidation combination. Treatment of the prochiral cyclohexadienone acid (these alkenes are enantiotopic) with bromine initiated a stereospecific reaction that resulted in a racemic mixture of bromolactones. Addition of hydroxide to the lactone led to a tetrahedral intermediate that collapsed, displacing bromide to give the α,β-epoxyketone. Repetition of the

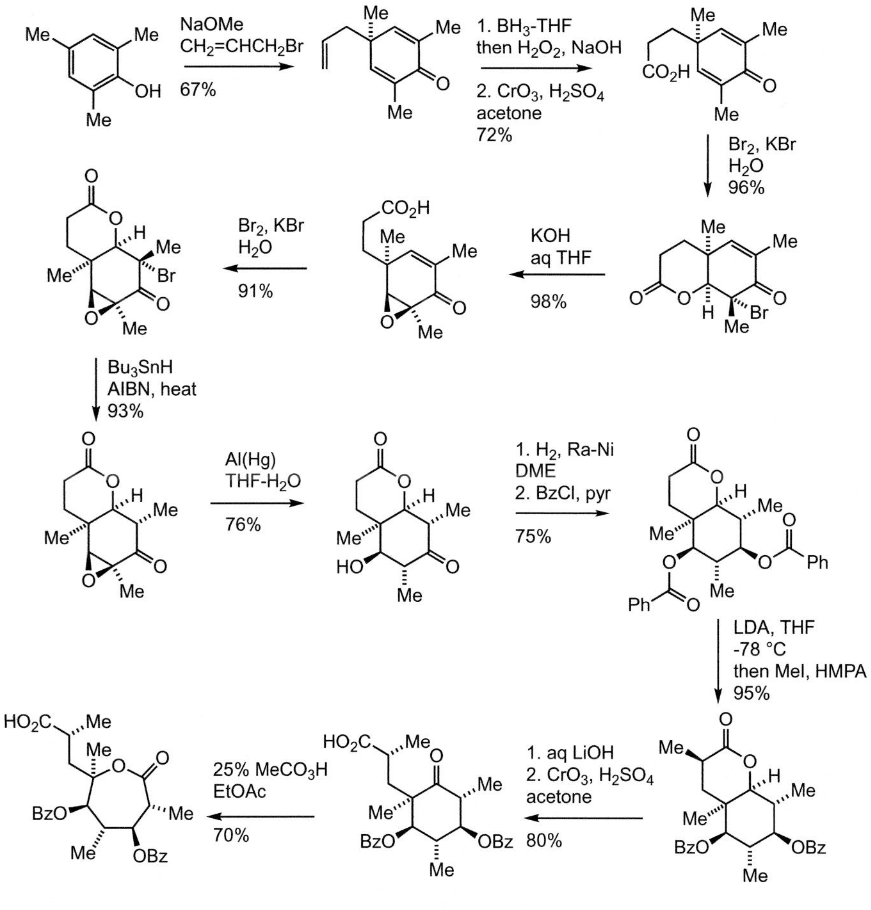

FIGURE 5.4. Corey's synthesis of the C1–C9 segment of erythronolide B.

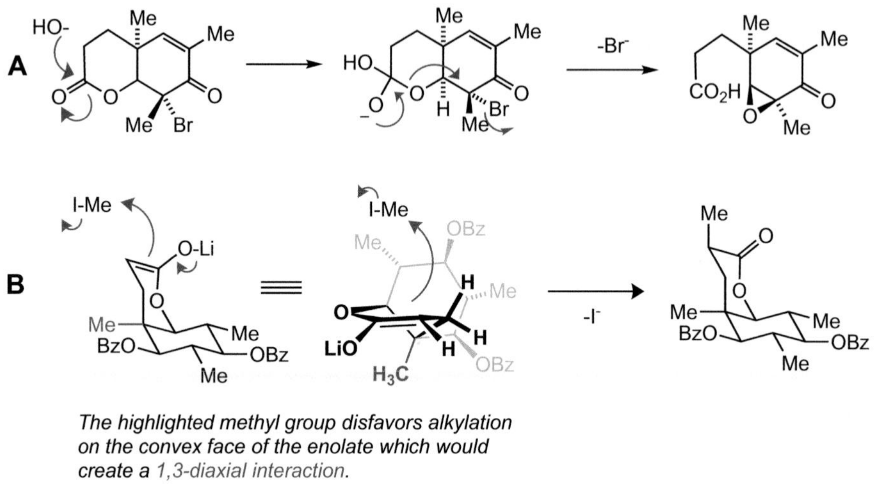

The highlighted methyl group disfavors alkylation on the convex face of the enolate which would create a 1,3-diaxial interaction.

FIGURE 5.5. Mechanistic rationales for two key reactions in Corey's synthesis of erythronolide B. (A) Stereospecific epoxide formation. (B) Stereoselective alkylation of a lactone.

bromolactonization on the remaining alkene led to a compound that has two C(=O)–C–X moieties (X = Br and epoxide) that are both susceptible to reductive cleavage of the C–X bond. The C–Br bond was cleaved first via a radical chain reaction that employed tributyltin hydride to quench the initially formed radical. The α,β-epoxyketone was then reduced with aluminum amalgam. You may ask why these two reductive cleavages couldn't be performed together with aluminum amalgam. The reason is that the intermediate enolate, formed by the addition of two electrons to the α-bromoketone, would likely lead to β-elimination of the lactone carboxylate. Contrast this with the β-alkoxyenolate formed by the addition of two electrons to the α,β-epoxyketone. Recall that the pKa of a carboxylic acid is approximately 4.5 and that of an alcohol is ~15, making the former a much better leaving group. Raney nickel was used to reduce the ketone to the more stable equatorial alcohol. Both alcohols were protected as benzoate esters in preparation for the next step. Deprotonation of the lactone with lithium diisopropylamide (LDA) at low temperature produced an enolate that was alkylated on the less hindered enolate face with methyl iodide. The lactone was then saponified, and the newly revealed alcohol oxidized to a ketone with Jones reagent. The stage was now set for the key Baeyer–Villiger reaction (see Corey's use of this reaction for prostaglandin synthesis in the previous chapter) that afforded a seven-membered lactone corresponding to C1–C9 of the target molecule. The resulting C1–C9 carboxylic acid is ready for coupling to the C10–C15 subunit. But first, the C1–C9 subunit had to be synthesized.

Synthesis of the C10–C15 portion of erythronolide B (Figure 5.6) began with nucleophilic epoxidation of crotonic acid followed by classical resolution of the racemate. The carboxylic acid was reduced, and the resulting epoxylalcohol was protected. The epoxide was opened regioselectively (attack at the carbon that can better

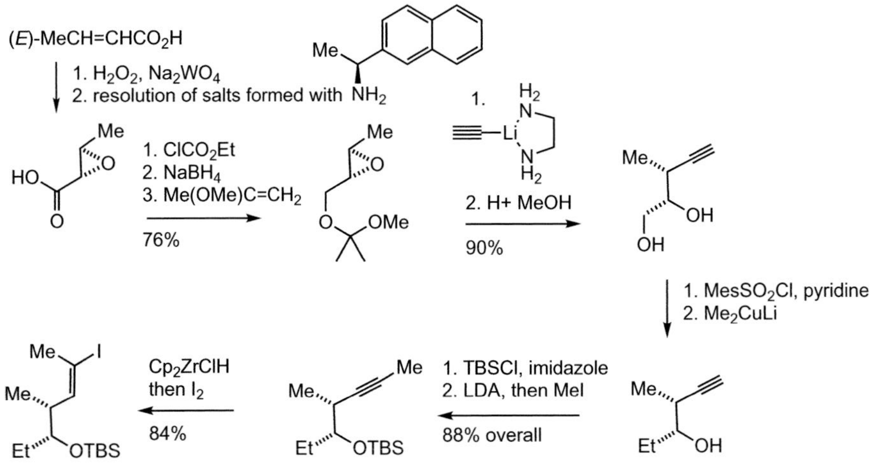

FIGURE 5.6.   Corey's synthesis of the C10–C15 portion of erythronolide B.

stabilize a partial positive charge) with a lithium acetylide, and the primary alcohol was transformed into a methyl group as described earlier. After protection of the alcohol, the monosubstituted acetylide was methylated and then subjected to a ste-reospecific cis-hydrozirconation-iodination sequence to give the vinyl iodide.

Completion of the erythronolide B synthesis (Figure 5.7) commenced with the conversion of the vinyl iodide to a Grignard reagent by treating the former with sec-butyllithium and then MgBr$_2$. The Grignard reagent reacted with the pyridinethiol ester prepared by reacting the C1–C9 carboxylic acid with 2,2'-dipyridyldisulfide and triphenylphosphine. This reaction proceeds through a tetrahedral intermediate that is stabilized by chelation at low temperature. Upon quenching with aqueous buffer at ambient temperature, unreacted Grignard reagent is rapidly decomposed, and the ketone is revealed. Because the Grignard component was enantiomerically pure and the thioester was racemic, a 1:1 mixture of diastereomers was obtained and carried on to the next step. The ketone was reduced stereoselectively with zinc boro-hydride (a fortuitus outcome that probably resulted from chelation of the zinc ion) to give the β-alcohol that underwent a spontaneous translactonization to give a ten-membered lactone ring. This compound was subjected to a battery of reactions that effected 1) desilylation, (2) opening of the lactone, (3) removal of the benzoate esters, (4) formation of a methyl ester (chromatographic separation of the diastereomers), (5) installation of an acetonide ring, (6) removal of an extraneous 2-methoxypropyl ether, and (7) saponification of the methyl ester to give the seco-acid.

Macrolactonization was accomplished using the dual activation methodology that Corey had developed separately. The acetonide ring played an important role in this entropy-disfavored reaction in that it locked part of the linear hydroxy acid into a conformation that favored macrocyclization. The synthetic finale began with che-moselective oxidation of the allylic C9 alcohol with MnO$_2$ to give an enone that was subjected to nucleophilic epoxidation. The observed selectivity can be rationalized

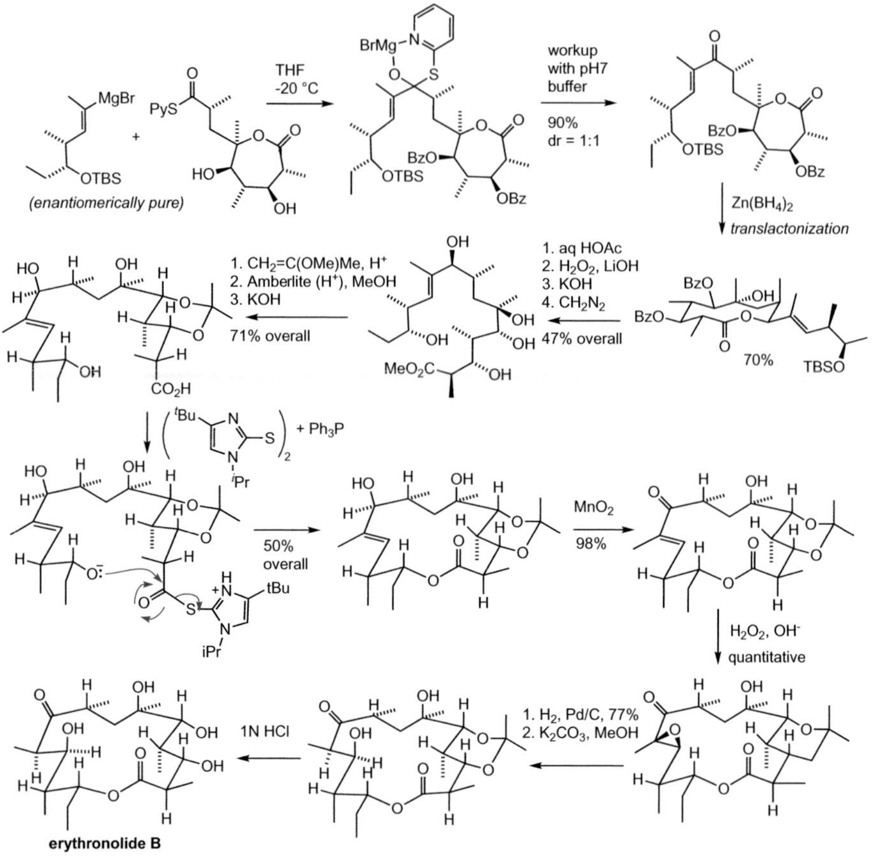

FIGURE 5.7. Union of the C1–C9 and C10–C15 units and completion of the erythronolide B synthesis.

by a conformation that places the enone functional group orthogonal to the macrocyclic plane, thus effectively blocking one face of the π-system via transannular steric interactions. The resulting epoxy ketone was cleaved reductively to give the aldol, and the C10 methyl group epimerized to the thermodynamically favored β-configuration. Finally, removal of the acetonide group produced erythronolide B.

Corey's synthesis of erythronolide B proceeded in 30 steps from 2,4,6-trimethylphenol and had a 33% ideality score. In addition to being the first successful synthesis of a stereochemically complex macrolide, it showcased Corey's ingenuity in devising a strategy that employed relatively simple reactions to solve a complex problem. Highlights included the sequential bromolactonizations and Baeyer–Villiger reaction to set the required C1–C6 stereochemistry and the use of an acetonide protecting group to restrict conformational mobility of the penultimate linear hydroxy-acid and facilitate the macrolactonization. On the other hand, a major efficiency problem was the need for a classical resolution to obtain the C10–C15 segment in

enantiomerically pure form and the production of an equimolar amount of an undesired diastereomer during the union of the racemic C1–C9 and enantiomerically
pure C10–C15 segments.

EPOTHILONE A

The development of Ru(I)-catalyzed olefin metathesis and asymmetric aldol meth-
odologies have provided alternative macrocyclization options augmenting the obvious macrolactonization strategy. This was nicely illustrated by three synthetic
approaches to our second target, the macrolide antibiotic epothilone A (Figure 5.8).
The epothilones are potential anticancer drugs that are isolated from soil-dwelling
myxobacterium *Sorangium cellulosum*. Like Taxol but with better efficacy and fewer
adverse effects, they act by binding tubulin, interfering with microtubule disassembly. This halts mitosis at the G2–M transition and leads to apoptosis (cell death).
These properties along with their simpler structures and difficulties associated with
fermentation of myxobacterium make the epothilones attractive targets for synthesis.

Our focus will be on the macrocyclizations developed by K. C. Nicolaou,[3] Samuel
Danishefsky,[4] Dieter Schinzer,[5] and Alois Fürstner.[6]

Formation of the 16-membered ring was first accomplished via a macrolactonization reaction (Figure 5.8, Path A). The Yamaguchi procedure (2,4,6-trichlorobenzoyl

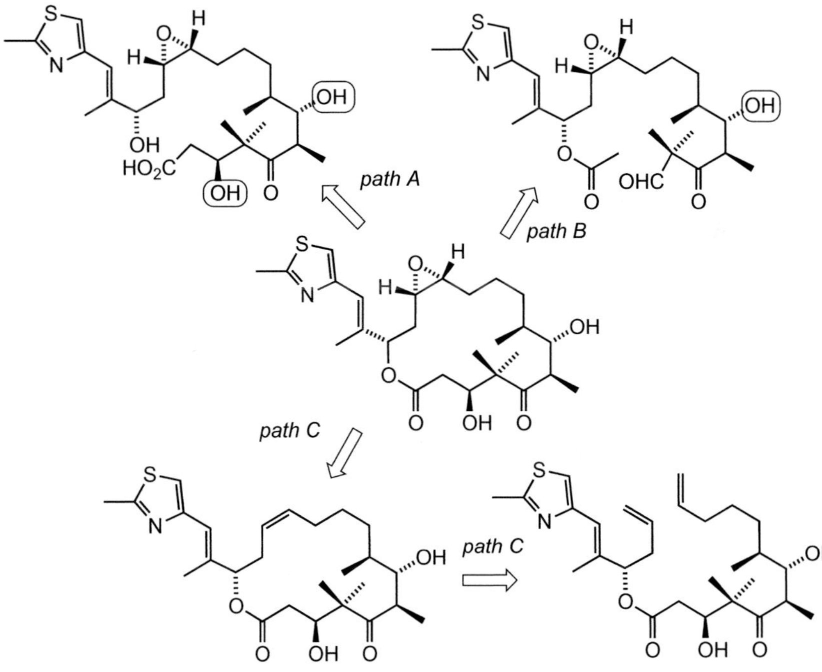

FIGURE 5.8. Macrocyclization strategies that have been applied to the synthesis of epothilone A.

chloride, Et_3N, DMAP/toluene, rt) was used for this macrocyclization. This acylation reaction may involve a mixed anhydride, an acyl pyridinium, and/or a ketene as a reactive intermediate. A mixed aldol retron is also present in epothilone A (Figure 5.8, Path B), and its unique structure could be exploited for macrocyclization, as the aldehyde component does not have any other α-protons, and only one enolate–aldehyde combination is possible. However, this disconnection may be considered rather risky, as aldol additions can be reversible, and it is not immediately obvious what the stereochemistry at C3 will be. A third disconnection (Figure 5.8, Path C) can be made once the C12–C13 alkene is revealed by an epoxidation retron. This alkene (itself a natural product: epothilone C) may be prepared by a ring-closing metathesis (RCM) reaction; though, again, it is not obvious what the alkene stereochemistry (cis or trans) will be. An added feature of this strategy is that by modifying one of the alkenes, the synthesis may be performed on a resin. Performing a synthesis on a solid support is advantageous in terms of product purification, as reagents and byproducts may be simply washed away (as is well known for peptides). The solid-phase synthesis of epothilone A would enable the rapid generation of analogues for biological screening.

Let's look at the metathesis-based synthesis of epothilone A, reported by the Nicolaou group, in more detail. We will analyze the synthesis from both retrosynthetic and synthetic directions. The retrosynthetic analysis (Figure 5.9) shows that the linear precursor may be cleaved at the C2–C3 bond to give a homoallylic alcohol and a syn-aldol. The homoallylic alcohol can be prepared in enantiomerically pure form using Brown's asymmetric allylation reagent (R* = (+)-Ipc, where Ipc is (+)-isopino-campheyl). The syn-aldol was synthesized by the union of a chiral (Z)-enolate and a chiral aldehyde via a Zimmerman–Traxler transition state. 2-Methylhept-6-enal was made by asymmetric alkylation on the Re face of the (Z)-enolate formed from a propionylated derivative of Oppolzer's camphorsultam (Figure 5.10).[7] The source of the stereocontrol in this chiral auxiliary mediated reaction is somewhat counterintuitive, as one might expect that one of the gem dimethyl groups would block the Re face of the (Z)-enolate. However, the sultam nitrogen is slightly pyramidalized moving the methyl group away from the enolate.

The details of Nicolaou's synthesis of epothilone A are shown in Figure 5.11. The β-hydroxy keto acid was formed by the Brown asymmetric allylation of 2,2-dimethyl-3-oxopentanal followed by oxidative processing of the vinyl group. However, the aldol addition reaction that formed the C6–C7 bond exhibited a low diastereomer ratio (dr). This was likely the result of mismatched stereocontrol elements in the two reaction partners. Application of Cram's model for nucleophilic additions to chiral aldehydes supports this hypothesis. Macrocyclic RCM proceeded in good yield with the Grubbs catalyst but gave a mixture of (Z)- and I-alkenes that were separated. The tert-butyldimethylsilyl (TBS) ether was removed with trifluoroacetic acid (TFA), and the resulting macrocyclic (Z)-alkene was epoxidized selectively to give epothilone A.

A Brown allylation was also used to prepare the thiazole containing alcohol (Figure 5.12). TI(E)-enal is prepared in good yield with a stabilized Wittig reagent. As expected, the 4-formylthiazole is more reactive toward the ylide than the more conjugated enal.

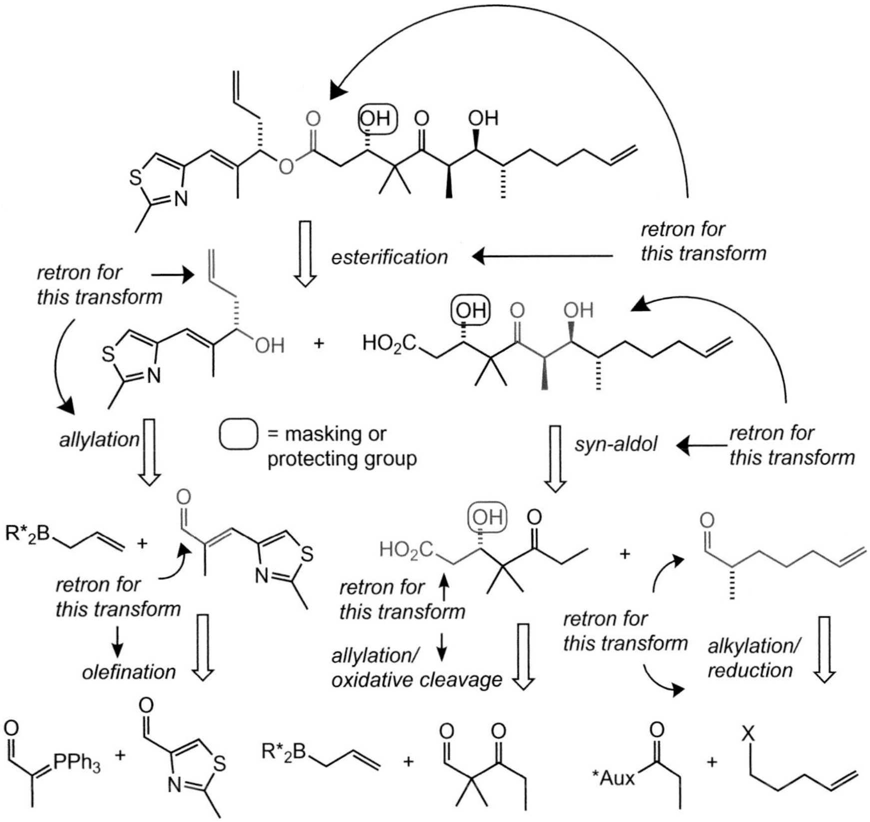

FIGURE 5.9. Retrosynthetic disconnections for Nicolaou's approach to epothilone A. (Retrons are colored magenta.)

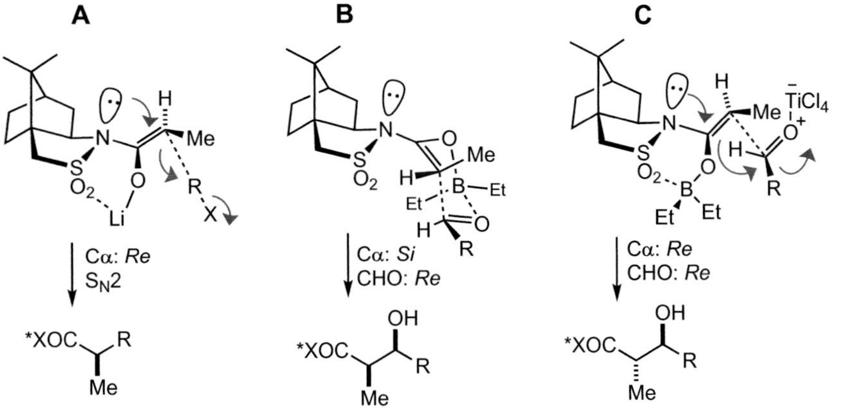

FIGURE 5.10. The use of Oppolzer's camphorsultam auxiliary for asymmetric A) alkylation, B) syn-aldol formation, and C) antialdol formation via chiral enolates.

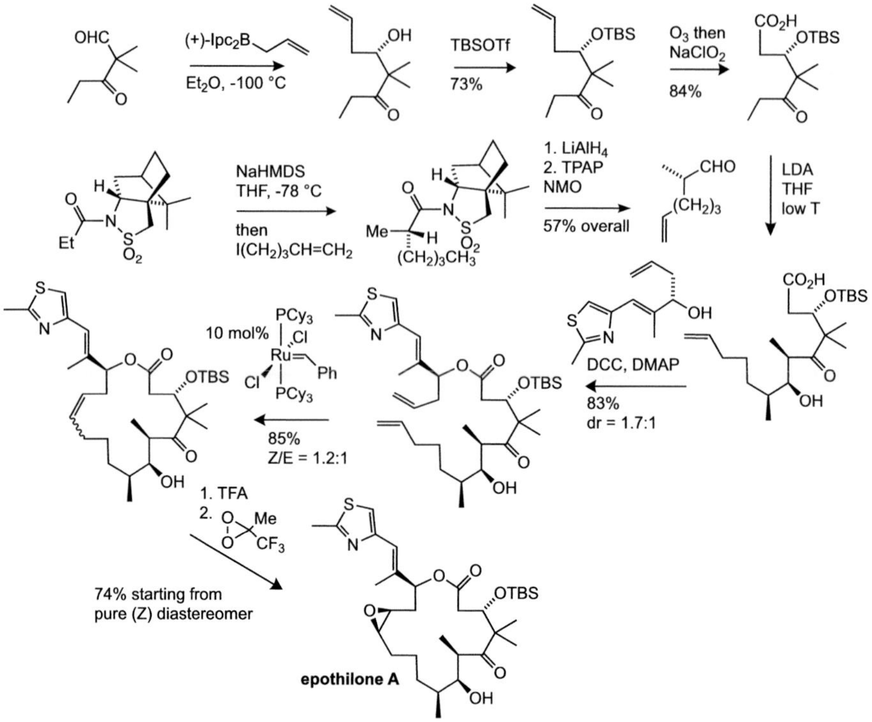

FIGURE 5.11. Nicolaou's synthesis of epothilone A featuring a macrocyclic RCM.

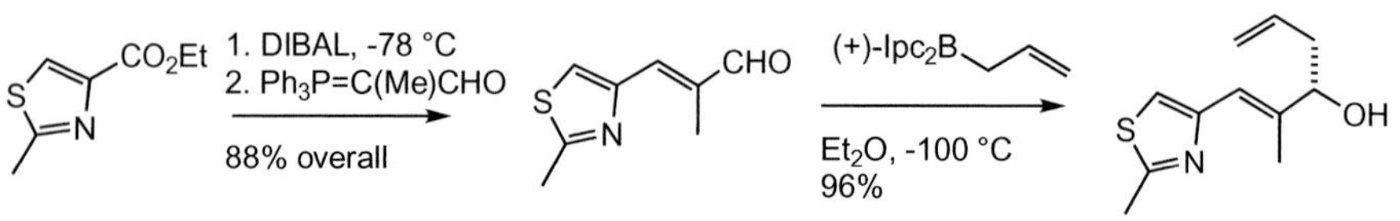

FIGURE 5.12. Synthesis of the thiazole containing metathesis partner.

The Nicolaou synthesis of epothilone A proceeded in eight steps from 2,2-dimethyl-3-oxopentanal (longest linear sequence) and had an ideality of 63%. Despite being quite efficient in terms of the number of steps, the low selectivities that were associated with the aldol reaction and RCM leave room for improvement. The problem attending the production of diastereomers was exacerbated in the solid phase synthesis of epothilone A because their separation must wait until the synthesis is complete and the products are released from the resin. In a clever move, Fürstner side-stepped the RCM selectivity issue by employing a molybdenum (III) catalyzed ring closing alkyne metathesis (RCAM) reaction to form the alkyne-containing macrocycle. Installation of the alkyne was followed by its semi-hydrogenation using a poisoned catalyst producing epothilone C (Figure 5.13). Because

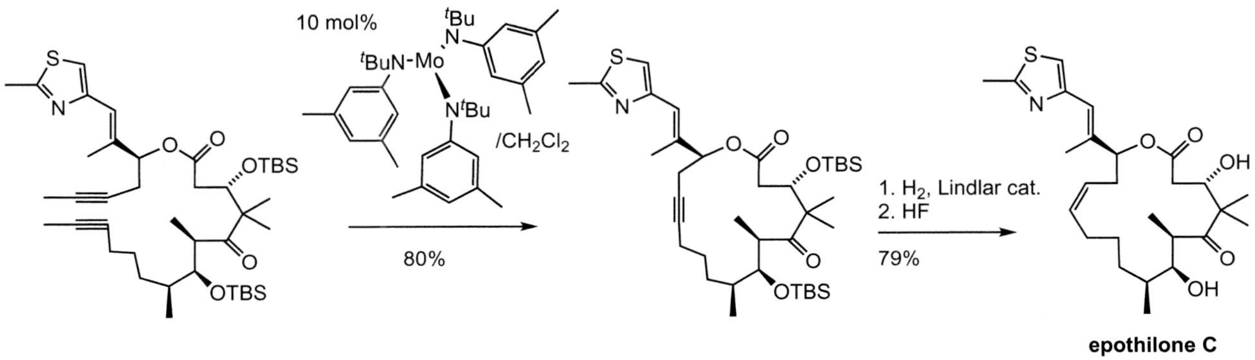

FIGURE 5.13. Fürstner's solution to the RCM selectivity problem.

epothilone C had been converted to epothilone A, this constituted a formal synthesis of epothilone A as well. With relatively straightforward synthetic approaches to the epothilone natural products in hand, recent efforts have been focused on developing more therapeutically promising unnatural epothilone analogues.

DISCODERMOLIDE

Our next example of a polyketide synthesis is the Novartis large-scale synthesis of discodermolide,[8] which is notable because it involves the total synthesis (rather than semi-synthesis) of an unmodified natural product that made it to the clinic. The natural product is obtained from a deep-water sponge (*Discodermia dissoluta*). Like Taxol and the epotholines, discodermolide showed anticancer potential due to microtubule stabilization. Because sufficient material for this trial could not be obtained from natural sources, total synthesis was used to solve the supply problem. Synthetic planning by Stuart Mickel and his team (Figure 5.14, retrons colored magenta) began with the opening of the lactone followed by a disconnection at the C6–C7 bond using an aldol transform. This produced a C1–C6 methyl ketone and a

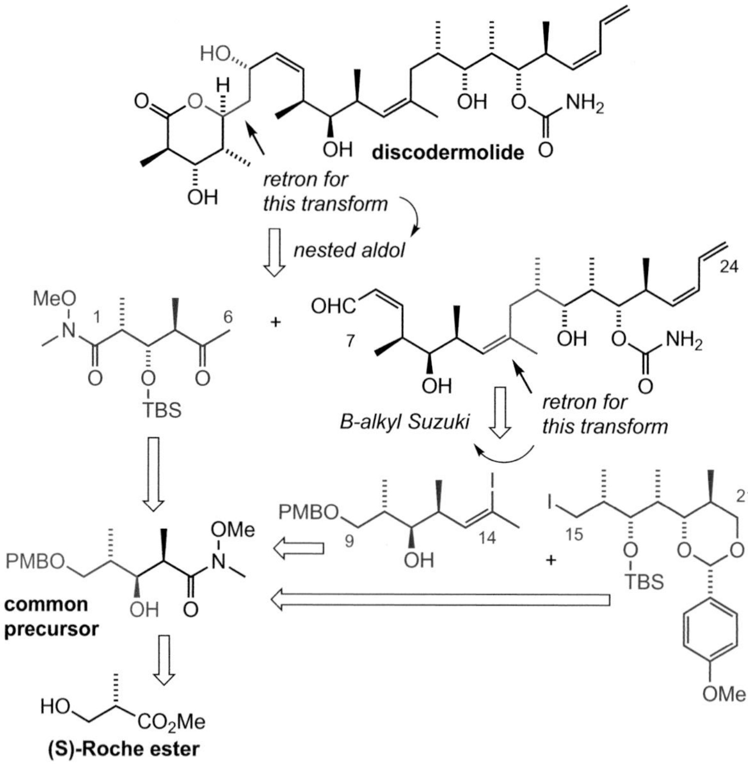

FIGURE 5.14. Mickel's retrosynthetic breakdown of discodermolide into three building blocks (colored blue) that come from a common precursor. The retrons are colored magenta.

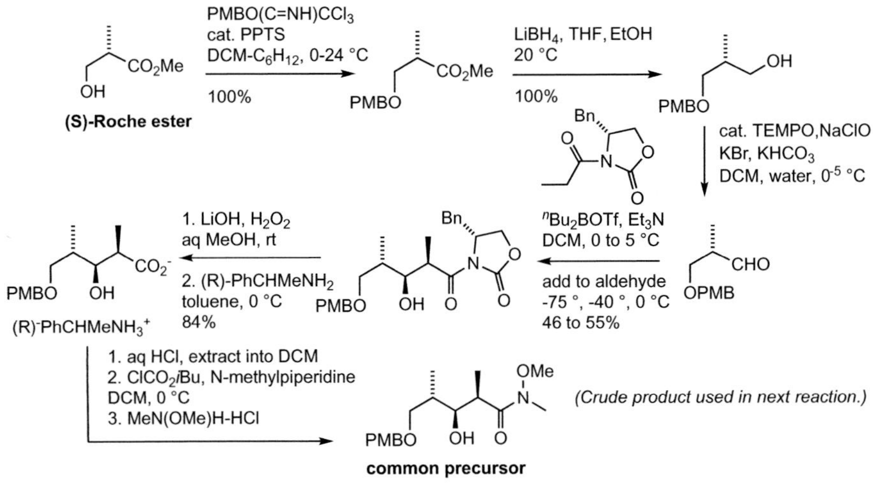

FIGURE 5.15. Synthesis of the common precursor to the discodermolide subunits.

C7–C24 aldehyde. The latter compound was subjected to a cross-coupling transform to give a vinyl iodide corresponding to C9–C14 and an alkyl iodide corresponding to C15–C24. The C1–C6, C9–C14, and C15–C24 subunits would all be derived from a common stereotriad precursor that was synthesized from the readily available (S)-Roche ester.

Synthesis of the common precursor (Figure 5.15) began with the protection of the alcohol as a p-methoxybenzyl ether. This protecting group was chosen for its versatility, as it can be removed by standard hydrogenolysis, oxidatively with 2,3-dichloro-5, 6-dicyano-1,4-benzoquinone (DDQ), and converted to a p-methoxybenzyl acetal. Next, the ester was converted to an aldehyde that was reacted with the (Z)-boron enolate of Evans's N-propionylated oxazolidinone to give the crystalline syn aldol. The chiral auxiliary was removed with lithium hydroperoxide (and recovered for reuse), and the acid was converted to a salt that enabled purification by recrystallization. The free acid was regenerated and converted to the versatile Weinreb amide, which can be converted directly to an aldehyde (hydride addition) or ketone (Grignard addition).

The Evans oxazolidinone auxiliaries have proven to be quite useful for the generation of chiral enolate equivalents.[9] To understand the observed stereoselectivity of the aldol addition, one must consider the enolate structure (E or Z) as well as the influence of the chiral auxiliary on the transition state (Figure 5.16). The (Z)-stereochemistry of the enolate minimizes allylic strain, as it adopts a conformation in which the dipoles of the auxiliary and the propionyl group are opposed. The aldol addition then proceeds through a chair-like Zimmerman–Traxler transition state that has the enolate attacking the Re face of the aldehyde and leads to a 2,3-syn configuration. However, the chiral aldehyde has its own preference for Si attack via a Felkin–Anh transition state. Which stereocontrol element will win the competition?

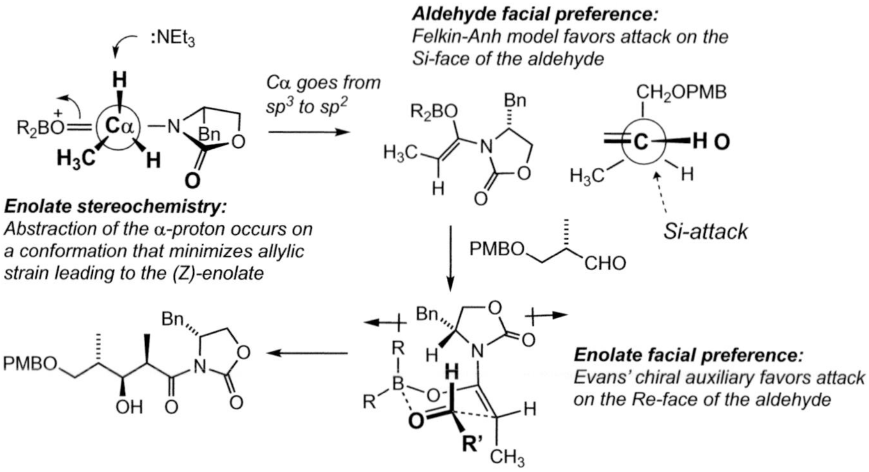

FIGURE 5.16. Rationale behind the stereoselectivity of the Evans aldol addition.

Fortunately, auxiliary stereocontrol is dominant, and the desired product is formed in good yield.

Synthesis of the C1–C6 subunit (Figure 5.17) commenced with removal of the para-methoxybenzyl (PMB) protecting group by palladium-catalyzed hydrogenolysis. The product was not isolated but treated with stoichiometric diacetoxyiodobenzene and a catalytic amount of 2,2,6,6-tetramethyl-piperidinyloxy (TEMPO), converting the primary alcohol to an aldehyde. This compound reacted with a Grignard reagent at the more reactive aldehyde carbonyl to give a mixture of alcohol diastereomers. Finally, Doering–Parikh oxidation of this mixture produced a ketone corresponding to the C1–C6 subunit that was isolated in good overall yield.

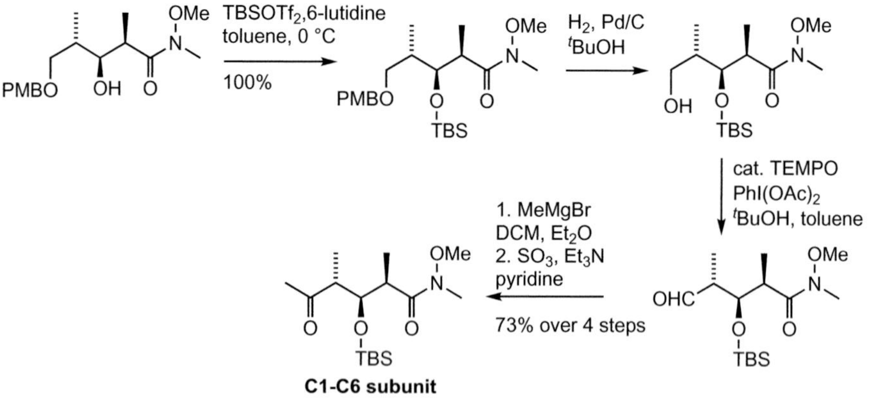

FIGURE 5.17. Synthesis of the C1–C6 subunit of discodermolide.

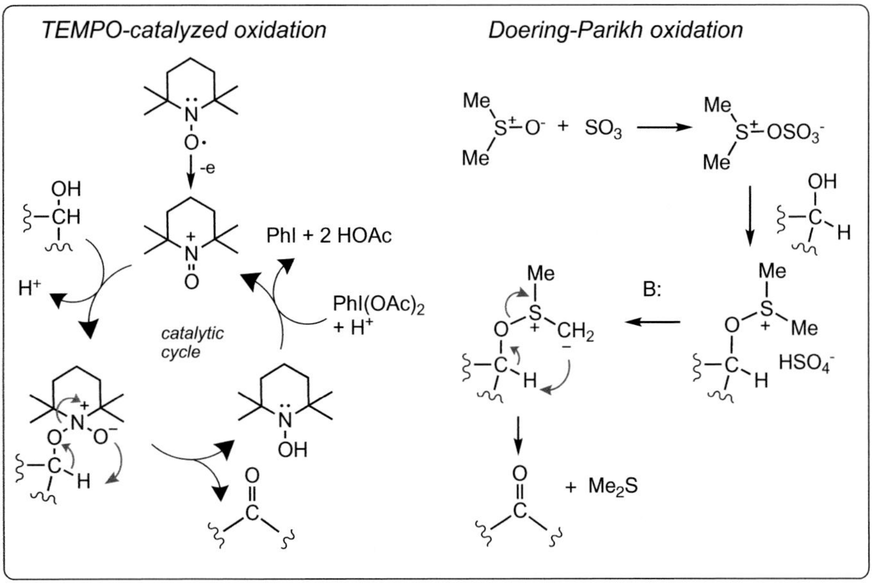

TEMPO-catalyzed oxidation   *Doering-Parikh oxidation*

The common precursor was converted to the C9–C14 subunit as follows (Figure 5.18). First, the alcohol was protected as a TBS ether. The Weinreb amide was converted to an aldehyde with Red-Al (Na$^+$ [(MeOCH$_2$CH$_2$O)$_2$AlH$_2$]$^-$), which forms a stable tetrahedral intermediate that does not collapse to a more reactive aldehyde until after the excess hydride is consumed during workup. The resulting aldehyde underwent a Wittig reaction with an unstabilized iodoethylidine ylide to give a

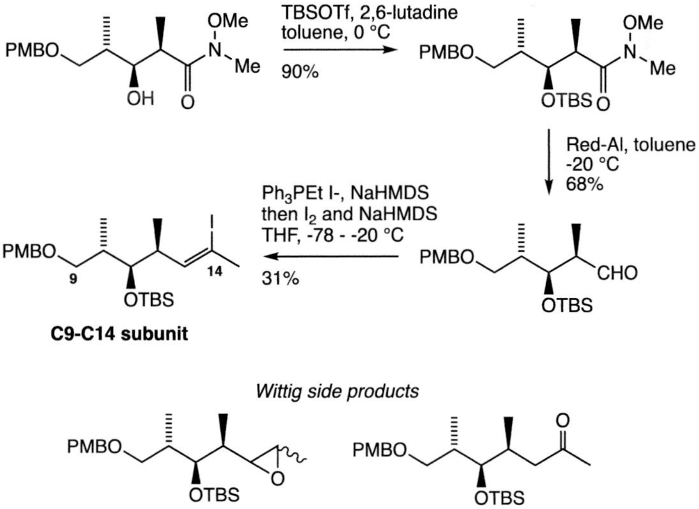

FIGURE 5.18. Synthesis of the C9–C14 subunit of discodermolide.

mixture favoring the (Z)-iodoalkene, which was isolated in 31% yield along with two byproducts. The epoxide could have resulted from displacement of iodide from an intermediate betaine followed by hydrolysis of the resulting alkyl phosphonium salt. The methyl ketone may have resulted from hydration of the product. Efforts to improve the yield of this reaction were unsuccessful.

Synthesis of the C15–C21 subunit (Figure 5.19) began with silylation of the alcohol. The imide was then reduced using lithium borohydride, releasing the Evans chiral auxiliary and producing a primary alcohol. This alcohol was converted to a primary iodide by a reagent Ph_3PI^+ I^- that was prepared *in situ* by the reaction of iodine with triphenylphosphine. With the three subunits in hand, all that remained to be done was to stitch them together and make some final functional group adjustments.

As shown in Figure 5.20, the C9–C14 and C15–C21 subunits were joined together using a B-alkyl Suzuki coupling reaction.[10] First, the alkyl iodide was converted to an alkyl lithium (via halogen–metal exchange) that reacted with 9-methoxy-9-borabicyclo[3.3.1]nonyl (BBN) to give a trialkyl borane (or its boronate salt). This route to the trialkylborane was likely chosen over hydroboration of a 15,16-alkene because the configuration at C16 was unambiguously set in the starting Roche aldehyde and the fact that it utilized the common precursor. This trialkylborane was treated with the vinyl iodide and a palladium pre-catalyst, resulting in the formation of the desired cross-coupling product in 73% yield. Turning to the other end of the

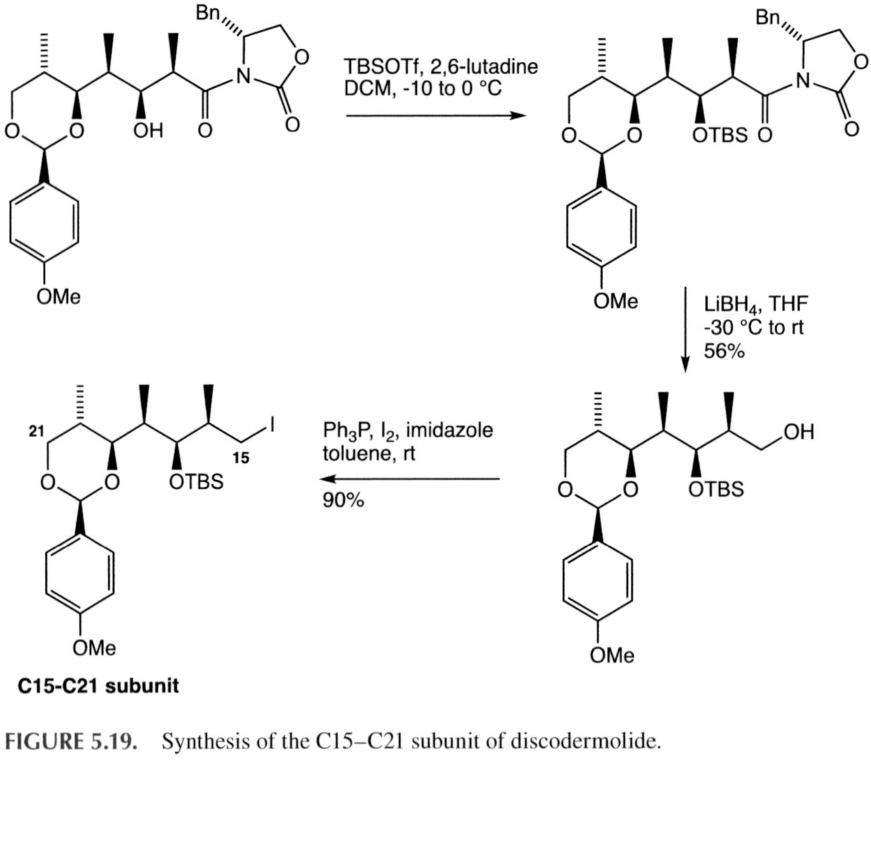

FIGURE 5.19.　Synthesis of the C15–C21 subunit of discodermolide.

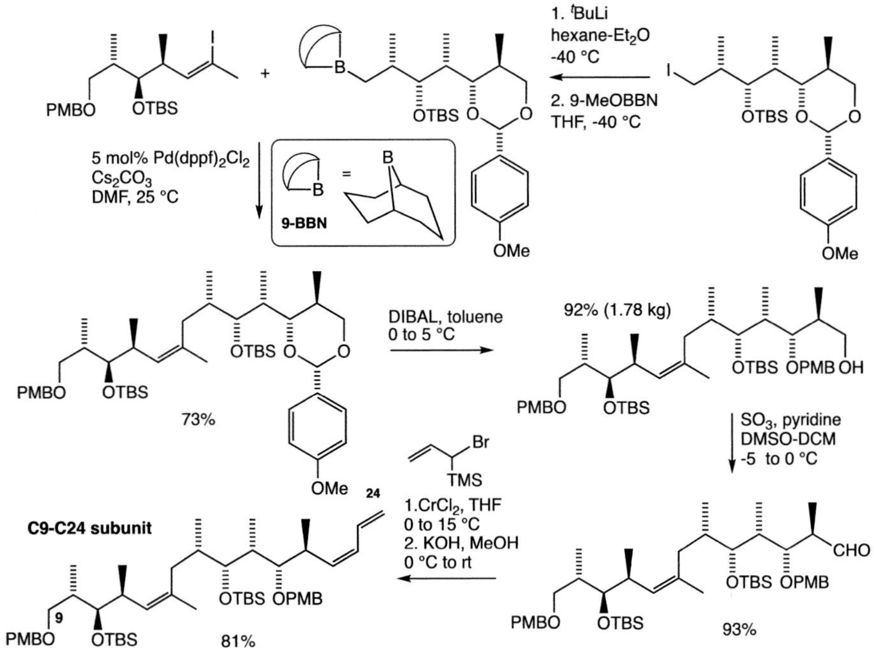

FIGURE 5.20. Synthesis of the C9–C24 subunit of discodermolide.

molecule, the p-methoxyphenyl acetal was regioselectively cleaved with diisobutylaluminum hydride (DIBAL) to give the 19-OPMB ether and a primary alcohol. After Doering–Parikh oxidation of the alcohol to an aldehyde, a silicon-modified stoichiometric Hiyama–Nozaki allylation reaction[11] using a trimethylsilyl substituted allyl bromide installed the C9–C21 subunit in 93% yield. The stereoselectivity of this allylation/elimination sequence can be accounted for (Figure 5.21) by an

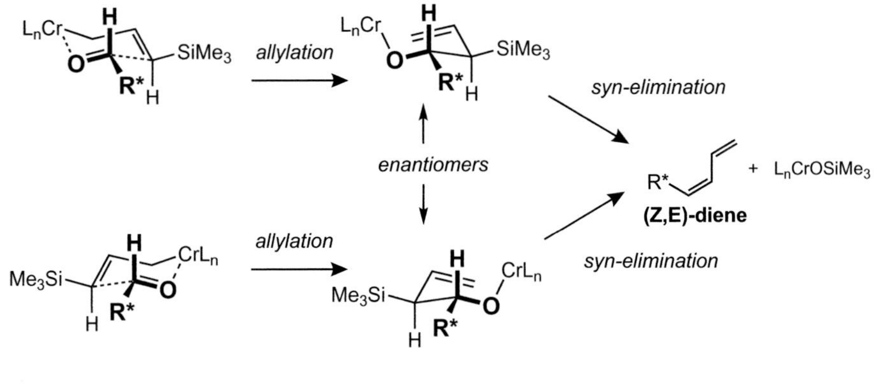

FIGURE 5.21. Mechanism of the silicon-modified Cr(II)-mediated allylation/elimination to form the (Z,E)-diene.

equilibrating allylchromium species that leads to a preferred chair-like Zimmerman–Traxler transition state followed by the syn-elimination of a siloxide reminiscent of the Peterson olefination. Note that the chiral aldehyde component results in a mixture of diastereomers that converge to give the same (Z, E)-diene.

In preparation for the final stage of the synthesis, a two-carbon subunit corresponding to C7 and C8 needed to be installed (Figure 5.22). First, both PMB ethers were removed using 2,3-dichloro-5,6-dicyano benzoquinone (DDQ), revealing a primary and secondary alcohol. The primary alcohol was oxidized to an aldehyde using the TEMPO-PhI(OAc)$_2$ reagent (leaving the free secondary alcohol untouched). The aldehyde was then subjected to a Still–Gennari Wittig olefination to give the (Z)-enoate. The urethane was attached to the free alcohol at C19 via its addition to an isocyanate. This was followed by reduction of the methyl ester to a primary alcohol using DIBAL. Note that, with certain substrates, the DIBAL reduction of esters proceeds all the way to the primary alcohol, even when the reaction is run at low temperatures.

The stage was now set for completing the discodermolide skeleton using acetate aldol chemistry that had been developed by Ian Paterson (Figure 5.23). This involved converting the methyl ketone of subunit C1–C6 into a chiral boron enolate by treating it with (+)-DIP-Cl and Et$_3$N. Reaction of this chiral enolate with the C7–C24 aldehyde resulted in a 63% yield of the desired (7S) aldol along with 23% of the (7R) epimer. The low diastereoselectivity (dr ~ 3:1) of this reaction is likely due to mismatched stereocontrol elements with the substrate favoring the (7R) epimer and the boron ligands favoring the (7S) epimer.

For the synthesis finale (Figure 5.24), the major aldol product was subjected to an Evans–Saksena reduction that installed the (5S) alcohol. Exposure of this compound to HCl resulted in the formation of the target's δ-lactone and concomitant removal of the silyl protecting groups to afford synthetic discodermolide.

Evans-Saksena reduction

Although the natural product did not make it through the clinical trials and get approved as a drug, the synthesis of discodermolide by the Novartis process group enabled the clinical trials and demonstrated that the total synthesis of a complex molecule could be performed on a very large scale. This effort produced 60 g of material for biological testing in 30 steps (27% ideality) from the readily available Roche ester. The strength of this synthesis was the successful integration (and optimization) of chemistry developed in multiple academic labs to achieve an important

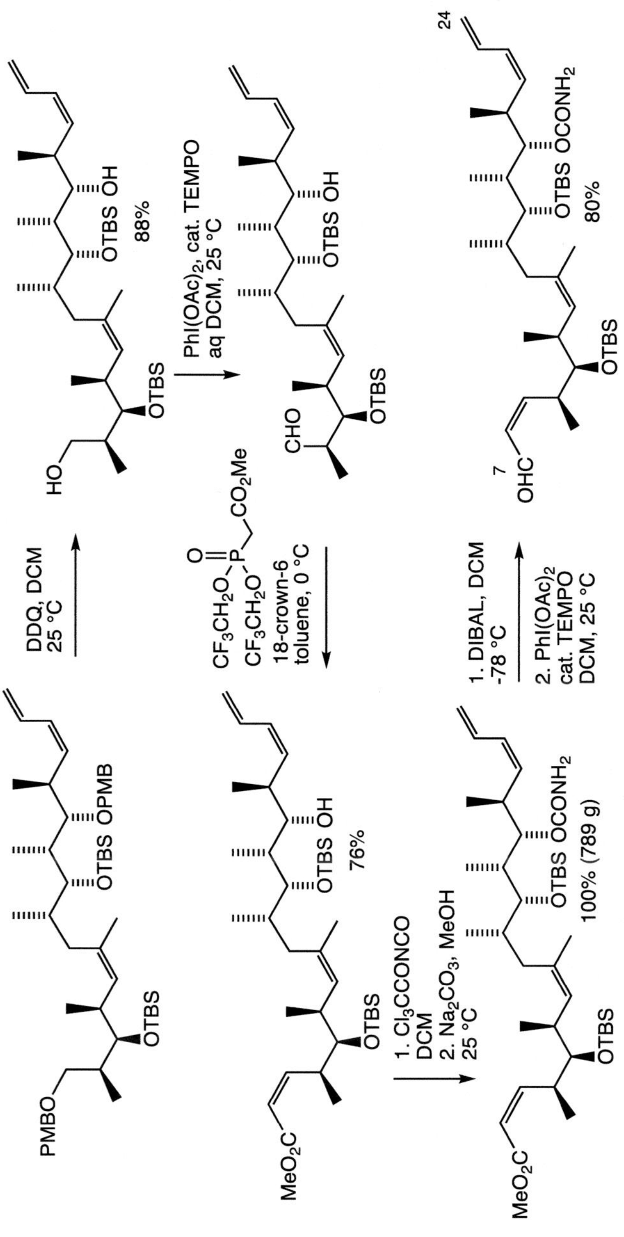

FIGURE 5.22. Synthesis of the C7–C24 subunit of discodermolide.

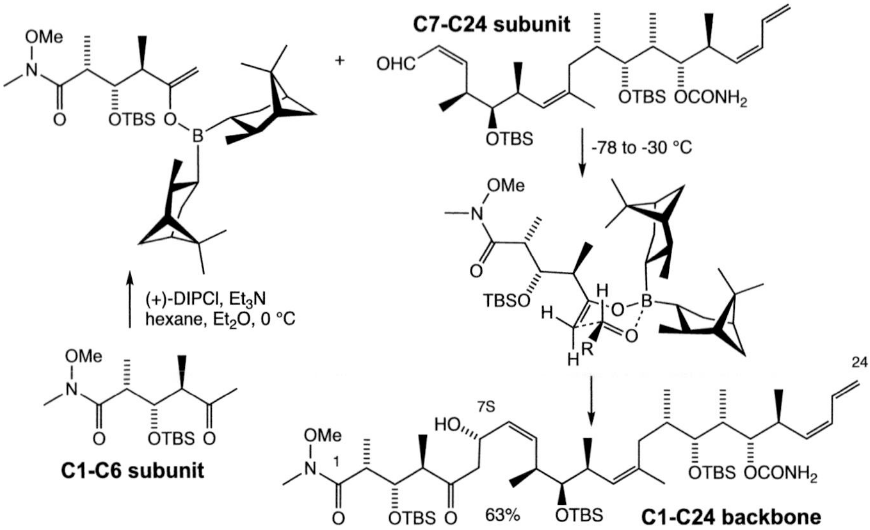

FIGURE 5.23. Merger of the subunits using Paterson's asymmetric aldol methodology.

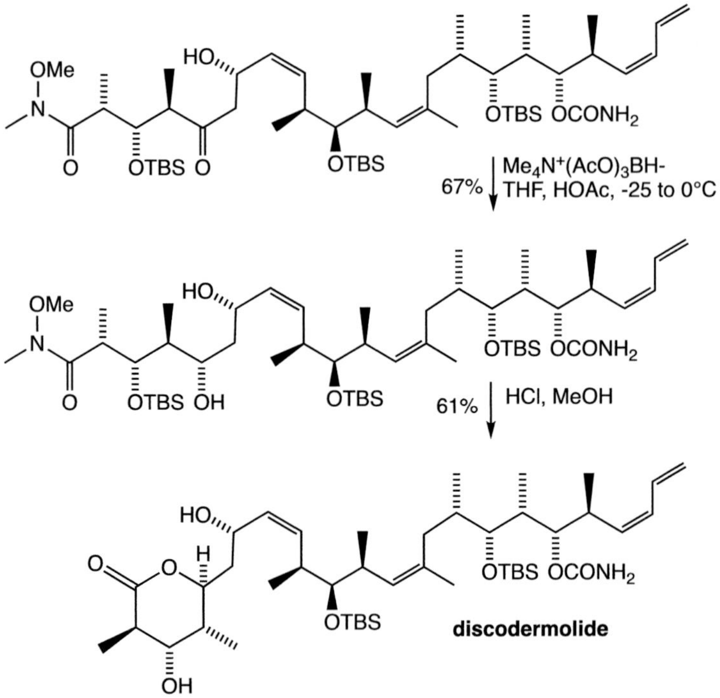

FIGURE 5.24. Synthetic finale and completion of the Novartis synthesis of discodermolide.

goal. As with any total synthesis, a variety of practical problems were encountered along the way. Most of these problems were solved. However, an intractable problem accompanied the Wittig reaction that was used to form the trisubstituted iodoalkene, wherein significant side product formation was observed.

BAHAMAOLIDE A

bahamaolide

Our next example of a polyketide synthesis targets bahamaolide A, a polyol macrolide antibiotic that was isolated from a Caribbean marine sediment sample. Its structure includes 11 carbon stereocenters (4,096 possible stereoisomers!), a conjugated hexaene, and a 36-membered lactone. Thus, bahamaolide A lays down the gauntlet for any synthetic chemist wishing to synthesize this natural product. The repeating 1,3-polyol motif in bahamaolide A provides a good platform for the discussion of iterative and bidirectional synthetic strategies. You are probably already familiar with iterative processes that are used to build polypeptides (repeating C–N bond formation) and nucleic acids (repeating P–O bond formation) in which the building blocks are amino acids and nucleotides, respectively. However, an iterative approach to 1,3-polyols is considerably more challenging, as it would not only involve C–C bond formation but also the introduction of a stereocenter at each iteration as well. An iterative approach that would use chemistry we have seen already includes the repetitive application of the three-step sequence: (1) Brown allylation, (2) alcohol protection, and (3) oxidative cleavage of the olefin, or (1) aldol addition of boron enolates or silyl enol ethers, (2) alcohol protection, and (3) carbonyl reduction. Thus, each iteration consists of three steps. A plan for the iterative synthesis of bahamaolide using either one of the two approaches just mentioned is presented in Figure 5.25. We will compare this linear approach to 1,3-polyols with one that is substantially different from it that involves the stereocontrolled iterative homologation of boronic esters to form the skeletal C–C bond rather than nucleophilic addition to an aldehyde. We will also see how symmetry can shorten a synthesis.

This novel approach to repeating 1,3-polyols was developed in the Aggarwal lab and applied to the synthesis of representative polyketides, including bahamaolide A.[12] The underlying chemistry is shown in Figure 5.26. Each iteration consists of two steps. The sequence begins with addition of a chiral carbenoid equivalent, ":C(Allyl)Bpin*" (where pin = pinacolate), to a primary alkyl boronic ester R^1CH_2Bpin. The resulting alkyl boronate undergoes stereospecific Matteson rearrangement with displacement of a 2,4,6-triisopropylbenzoate leaving group to install a boronic ester moiety at C1.

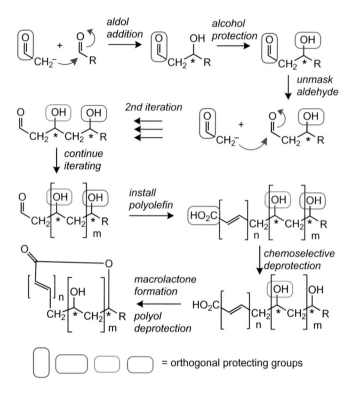

FIGURE 5.25. Linear approach to polyol macrolides utilizing either aldol additions or allyl borane additions to make the skeletal C–C bonds that link the repeating subunits.

The (ortho) isopropyl groups function to inhibit nucleophilic attack of the ester carbonyl and prevent directed metalation of the aromatic ring. In essence, the carbene synthon is formally inserted into the C–B bond stereoselectively. This homologation reaction is followed by a platinum-catalyzed asymmetric diboration that installs boronic esters at C3 and C4. The next iteration begins with chemoselective homologation of the primary boronic ester at C4, leaving the more hindered boronic ester at C3 intact. Repeating the process yields $R^1(CHBpinCH_2CHBpin)_nCH_2CHBpinR^2$ where the Bpin moieties are masked alcohols, all of which can be unmasked together at a late stage in the synthesis by oxidative rearrangement. Thus, boron not only actuates the key homologation mechanistically but also eliminates the need to install a protecting group with each iteration.

    The chiral carbenoid equivalent takes the form of a metalated benzoate ester, the pure enantiomers of which are readily prepared from their diastereomeric sulfoxide precursors. The development of enantiopure, bench-stable carbenoid building blocks that undergo metalo-boron exchange followed by stereospecific Matteson rearrangement was a critical requirement for this project. Treatment of these organolithium species with Andersen's reagent produced diastereomeric sec-alkyl boronates.

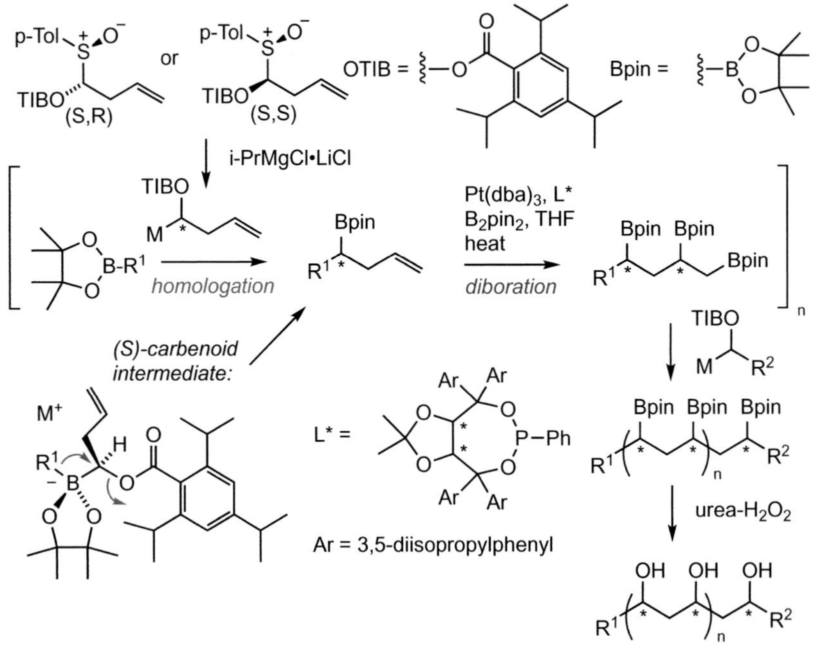

FIGURE 5.26. Iterative synthesis of repeating 1,3-polyols.

Aggarwal's application of this technology in the form of a 14-step synthesis of bahamaolide A is illustrated (via a combined retrosynthetic and synthetic format) in Figure 5.27. The overall synthetic strategy is instructive, as it not only introduces important boronic ester chemistry but also blends both retrospective and prospective thinking. The final stages (endgame) of the resulting synthesis are straightforward and use chemistry that should be familiar: introduction and removal of acetonide protecting groups, a Ru(I)-catalyzed cross metathesis reaction, Horner–Wadsworth–Emmons olefination, Yamaguchi macrolactonization, and functional group deprotection. Note that two different silyl ethers are employed, one being more labile than the other to facilitate the formation of the natural product's 36-membered macrolactone ring. Things get more interesting when one makes C–C bond disconnections so that one of the advanced intermediates (the octaboronic ester) has C2 symmetry. This property enables one to build the molecule in two directions simultaneously, generating two C–C bonds in each step. For the bahamaolide A synthesis, the termini must be differentiated with appropriate "Western" and "Eastern" capping modules. The Eastern cap was attached first. Not surprisingly, a statistical mixture of monosubstituted, disubstituted, and starting material was obtained. Attachment of the Western endcap was not problematic.

Synthesis of the repeating 1,3-polyol building block as well as the Eastern and Western end cap building blocks is shown in Figure 5.28. Benzoate directed deprotonation of the allyl benzoate using butyllithium complexed with a tetramethyl

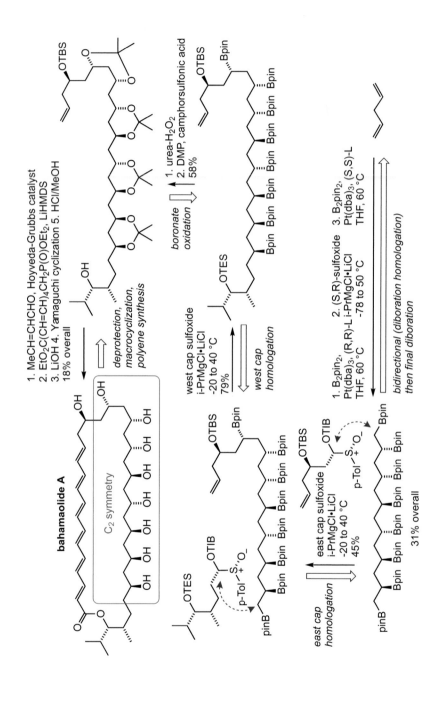

FIGURE 5.27.   Aggarwal's synthesis of bahamaolide A.

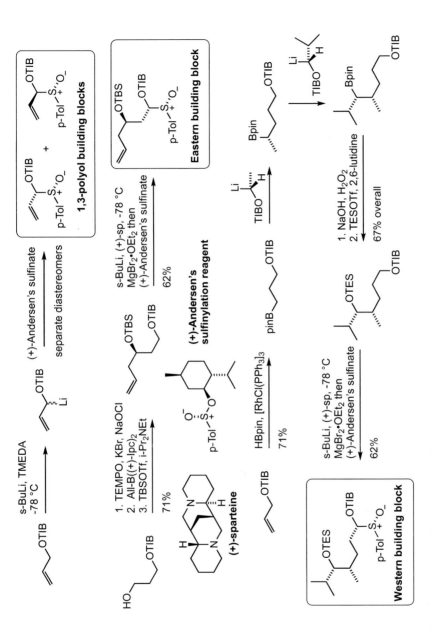

FIGURE 5.28. Syntheses of the chiral α-sulfinyl ethyl benzoate carbenoid precursors.

ethylene diamine (TMEDA) produced a racemic mixture of organolithium species. (+)-Sparteine could also be used as the diamine in this reaction, but, even though this compound is enantiomerically pure, it did not produce enantiomerically pure diastereomers. However, reaction of the racemic organolithium species with Andersen's sulfinylation reagent produced a separable mixture of enantiomerically pure diastereomers. These bench-stable carbenoid precursors were used for the homologation reaction. Synthesis of the Eastern building block began with an enantioselective Brown allylation followed by protection of the alcohol as a TBS ether then directed metalation and introduction of the α-sulfinyl group as described above. The Western building block was synthesized starting with the rhodium-catalyzed hydroboration of an allyl benzoate followed by homologation with enantioenriched lithium carbenoids to install the isopropyl and methyl substituents. Boronic ester oxidation produced an alcohol that was protected as a triethylsilyl (TES) ether that can be removed in the presence of a more stable TBS ether prior to macrolactonization.

Aggarwal's 14-step (longest linear sequence) synthesis of bahamaolide had an ideality of 75%. The polyol domain of the target was assembled in an iterative fashion using a modified version of the asymmetric Matteson reaction to install each "pseudoacetate repeat unit" with the correct configuration. The presence of local C2 symmetry in the polyol domain was taken advantage of, which enabled bidirectional homologation and enhanced efficiency. Because the intermediate boronate esters mask the target's secondary alcohols, there is no need for additional protecting groups. The result is an innovative and efficient synthesis of a complex macrolide.

ERIBULIN

We end this chapter with the production scale synthesis of the antitumor drug eribulin.[13] Eribulin is actually a truncated analog of the marine polyether macrolide halichondrin B, a natural product that is isolated from a marine sponge, *Halichondria okadai,* found off the coast of Japan (Figure 5.29). Therapeutic interest in this natural product began with the fact that halichondrin B exhibited extraordinary activity against Taxol-resistant metastatic breast cancer as well as liposarcoma. Its mode of action involves binding to tubulin, which inhibits the assembly of microtubules and leads to cell cycle arrest at the G2–M phase. The limited availability of halichondrin B from its natural source (7 mg of halichondrin B per kg of sponge, likely produced by a bacterial symbiant that resides on the sponge) resulted in a joint effort by academic and industrial laboratories (Yoshito Kishi's lab at Harvard and Eisai Pharmaceuticals in Japan) to develop a practical synthesis of this substance. However, its molecular size and complexity argued against the natural product itself as a potential drug but, rather, for identification of the pharmacophore (the portion of a molecule that is responsible for its bioactivity). Medicinal chemistry efforts resulted in the design of a viable analogue, eribulin (sold under the trade name Halavin), that was two-thirds the size of halichondrin B but had similar bioactivity. Still, with a molecular weight over 700, a sophisticated array of functionality, eight heterocyclic rings, and 19 stereocenters, the practical synthesis of this molecule was a formidable challenge.

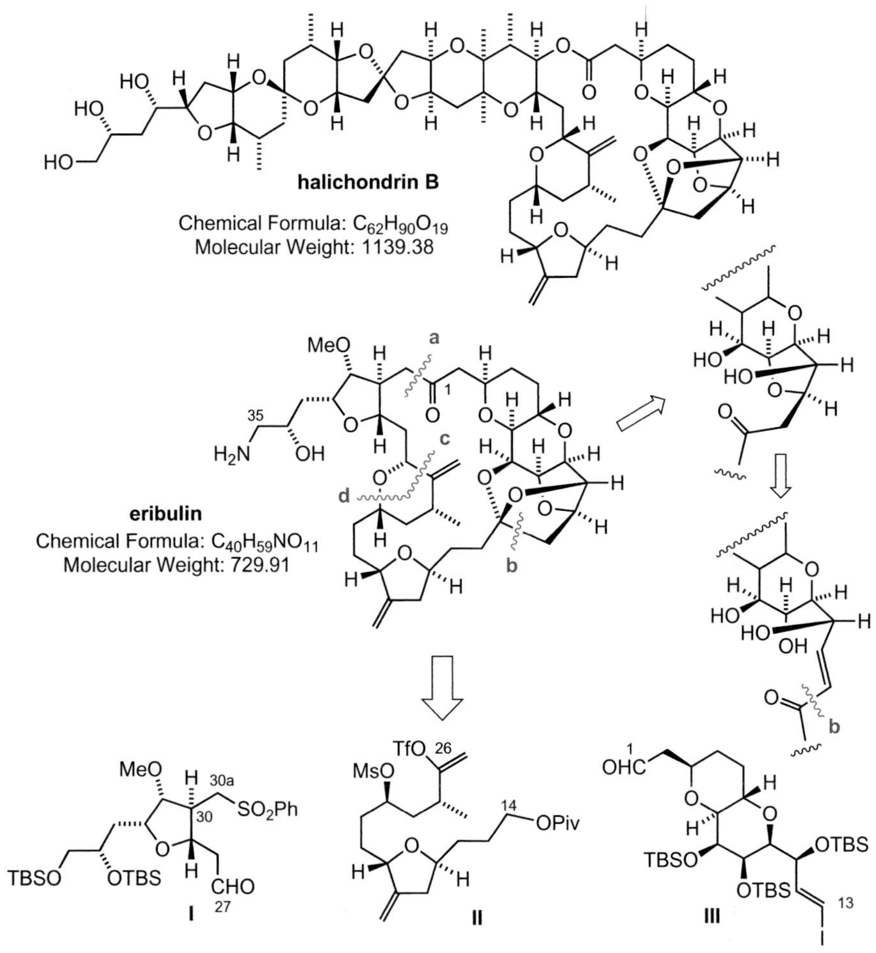

FIGURE 5.29. Molecular structures of the natural product halichondrin and the anticancer drug eribulin along with the key retrosynthetic disconnections leading to the three building blocks **I**, **II**, and **III**.

Retrosynthetic analysis of the strategy used to synthesize eribulin begins with four key primary bond disconnections that lead to the three (still quite complicated) building blocks **I**, **II**, and **III** shown. Disconnection "a" is relatively straightforward in that it keys for the net acylation of a methylene unit. As it turns out, this is accomplished via a nested transform involving a Julia reaction that forms a bond between C30a of building block **I** and C1 of building block **III**. The rationale for disconnection "b" is not so obvious but is revealed only after imaginary hydrolysis of the ketal moiety and β-elimination of an alkoxide moiety. Thus, the hidden transform involves the acylation of a vinyl nucleophile that forms a bond between C13 of building block **III** and C14 of building block **I**. Bond disconnection "c" also leads to a vinyl nucleophile adding to a carbonyl, foming a bond between C26 of building block **II** and C27 of building block **I**, but the intermediate alkoxide is also poised to undergo Williamson ether formation generating a 2-methylenetetrahydro-2*H*-pyran ring. While it is tempting to propose that one could use vinyl Grignard or vinyl lithium reagents as nucleophiles, one must also recognize that these reactions would be employed on highly functionalized substrates at late stages of the synthesis. Because of the basicity of Grignard and organolithium reagents, this could have a negative impact on chemoselectivity and stereoselectivity. New methodology, that has come to be known as the Nozaki–Hiyama–Kishi or NHK coupling reaction,[14] was developed to address these issues. The NHK reaction has been used in many synthetic contexts.

The NHK story is an interesting and instructive lesson in methodology development. It began with Nozaki and Hiyama's report of the Cr(II)-mediated allylation of aldehydes. The procedure involved generation of an allylchromium species *in situ* by reacting $CrCl_3$ with $LiAlH_4$ in the presence of allyl chloride and an aldehyde. Though this addition reaction was not very stereoselective when the aldehyde was chiral, it proceeded under mild conditions and tolerated a variety of functional groups. It was not long before vinylic halides were tried as substrates. However, the reaction of Cr(II) solutions generated by the $LiAlH_4$ reduction of Cr(III) salts with vinyl halides was found to be irreproducible and highly dependent on the batch of $CrCl_3$ that was used. A little detective work revealed that the addition of a catalytic quantity of $NiCl_2$ to the reaction mixture resulted in the desired addition regardless of the batch of Cr(III), indicating that certain batches of commercial $CrCl_3$ were contaminated with Ni(II) salts. The next problem to be tackled was how to make the NHK reaction enantioselective. Building on Fürstner's work on the catalytic NHK reaction, Kishi's group developed a set of chiral ligands for the enantioselective NHK reaction. The ligands not only resulted in stereocontrol but also rate acceleration. Three variations of the catalytic asymmetric NHK reaction are shown in Figure 5.30. The proposed mechanism for Variant **B** is also shown. The NHK allylation (Variant **A**) may actually proceed by multiple mechanisms as evidenced by the fact that this reaction does not depend on the presence of Ni(II) and evidence that supports a radical mechanism.

Turning next to the synthesis of building block **I** (Figure 5.31), the route developed by Kishi for his halichondrin B synthesis was followed. Readily available D-glucurono-3,6-lactone acetonide was deoxygenated by converting the hydroxyl group to a chloride followed by Pd-catalyzed hydrogenolysis. The lactone moiety was partially reduced to an aldehyde with DIBAL at low temperature. Peterson olefination followed by protection of the free alcohol produced an allyl substituted tetrahydrofuran that was subjected to Sharpless asymmetric dihydroxylation. After protection of the resulting vicinal diol as benzoate esters, the acetonide was removed with a titanium (IV) Lewis acid, and the resulting oxocarbenium ion reacted with allyltrimethylsilane. This allylation produced a compound with a free alcohol that was subjected to a Swern oxidation, and the resultant ketone was converted to an α,β-unsaturated sulfone with a Horner–Wadsworth–Emmons reagent. The benzyl ether was removed with trimethylsilyl iodide (TMSI). Hydroxyl-directed reduction

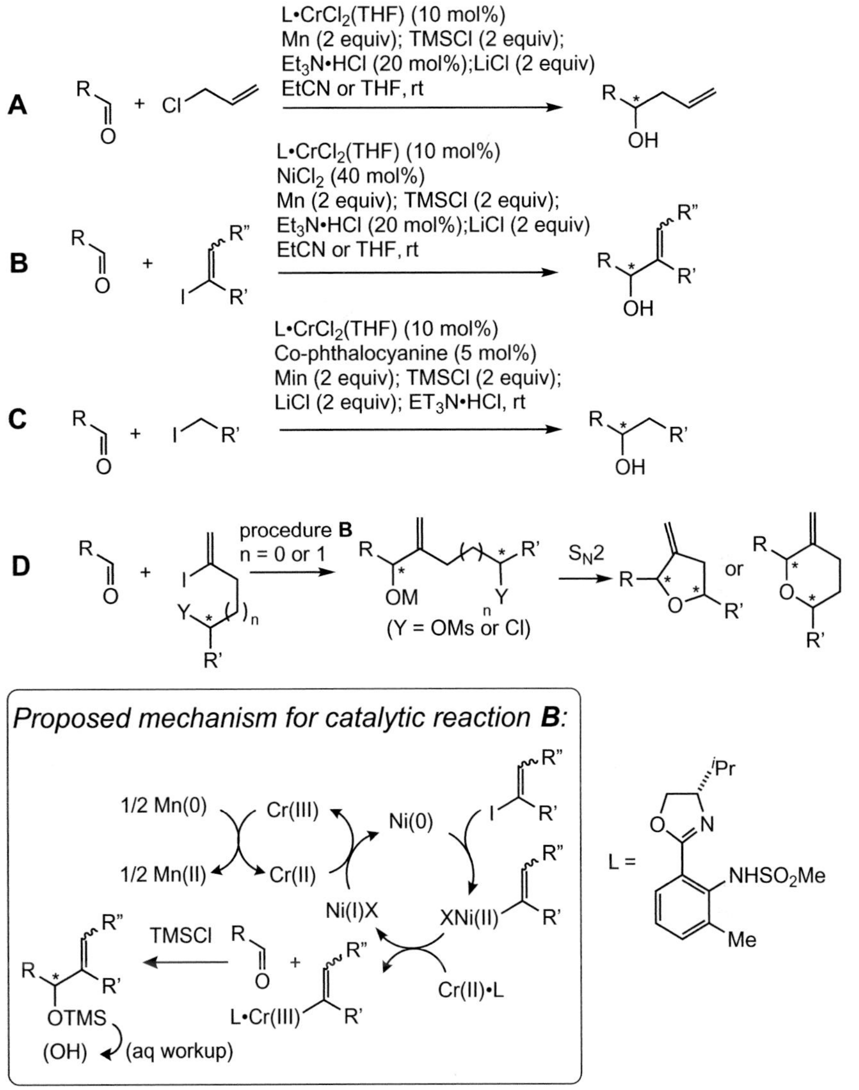

FIGURE 5.30. Three variations of the asymmetric catalytic NHK reaction: A) NHK allylation, B) NHK vinylation, C) NHK alkylation, and D) the combination of **B** with stereospecific cyclization. The proposed mechanism for Variant **B** is also shown.

of the electron-deficient olefin with triacetoxyborohydride occurred on the α-face and produced a tetrasubstituted tetrahydrofuran with the desired stereochemistry. Conversion of the vicinal benzoate protecting groups to a base stable acetonide and methylation of the remaining free alcohol introduced the requisite methyl ether. Finally, the acetonide was exchanged for two TBS ethers, and the allyl group was ozonized with a reductive workup to give building block **I**.

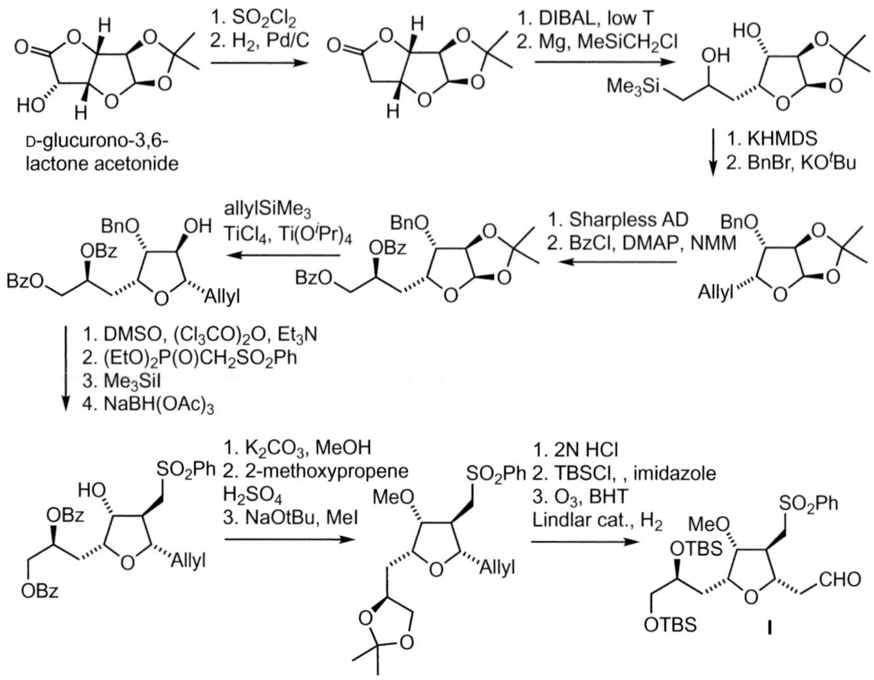

FIGURE 5.31.   Synthesis of building block **I**.

The synthesis of building block **II** (Figure 5.32) began with the (R)-epoxide, which was obtained in enantiomerically enriched form by hydrolytic kinetic resolution of the racemate.[15] Opening of the epoxide with the anion of dimethylmalonate produced an alkoxide that cyclized to give the γ-lactone. This compound was decarboxylated and then alkylated from the less hindered α-face via the lithium enolate. The γ-lactone was converted to a Weinreb amide, and the free alcohol protected as a TBS ether. The terminal olefin was then converted to an aldehyde corresponding to carbons 20–26 by dihydroxylation with osmium tetroxide followed by cleavage of the vicinal diol with sodium periodate. This aldehyde was coupled to a vinyl bromide corresponding to carbons 14–19 that was prepared from dihydrofuran (see Practice Problem 5), employing NHK Variant **B**. The initially formed hydroxy tosylate was exposed to mildly acidic silica gel that induced cyclization to a 3-methylenetatrahydrofuran. The Weinreb amide was then converted to a methyl ketone with methyl magnesium chloride at 0 °C. The kinetic enolate was formed at -70 °C and trapped with a bis-trifluoromethylsulfonyl imide. Both silyl ether protecting groups were removed with 6N HCl. The primary alcohol was selectively protected as a pivolate ester, and the secondary alcohol was converted to a mesylate completing the synthesis of building block **II**.

The synthesis of building block **III** from D-(-)-gulono-1,4-lactone (Figure 5.33) began with the formation of a bis-ketal. This was followed by partial reduction of the

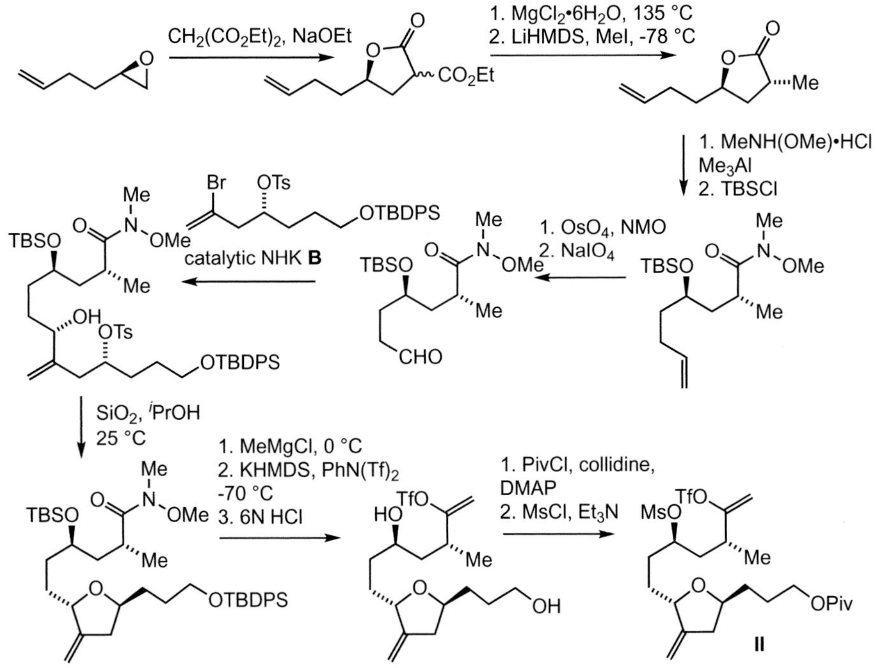

CH$_2$(CO$_2$Et)$_2$, NaOEt

1. MgCl$_2$•6H$_2$O, 135 °C
2. LiHMDS, MeI, -78 °C

CO$_2$Et

Me

1. MeNH(OMe)•HCl
   Me$_3$Al
2. TBSCl

Me
Br   OTs
TBSO
O   N   OMe
OTBDPS
Me
catalytic NHK **B**

Me
1. OsO$_4$, NMO
2. NaIO$_4$
TBSO
O   N   OMe
Me

Me
TBSO
O   N   OMe
Me

OH   OTs
OTBDPS

TBSO
O   N   OMe
Me
CHO

SiO$_2$, ^{i}PrOH
25 °C

Me
TBSO
O   N   OMe
1. MeMgCl, 0 °C
2. KHMDS, PhN(Tf)$_2$
   -70 °C
3. 6N HCl
Me
OTBDPS

1. PivCl, collidine,
   DMAP
2. MsCl, Et$_3$N

TfO
HO
Me
OH

TfO
MsO
Me
OPiv

II

FIGURE 5.32. Synthesis of building block **II**.

lactone to give a lactol that was in equilibrium with a hydroxy aldehyde which reacted with a methoxymethylene phosphonium ylide to give a mixture of methyl vinyl ethers. The sequence included four stereoselective reactions that deserve some additional explanation. Following an empirical model proposed by Kishi and coworkers in 1983 (Figure 5.34A) that generated OsO$_4$ *in situ* and underwent diastereoselective addition to the Re face of the alkene with the reagent approaching the double bond anti to the allylic C–O bond. In this reaction, the developing stereochemistry was linked to the substrate's configuration and optimal orbital overlap, passing through a conformation that minimized allylic strain. The resulting hemiacetal cyclized to the lactol that was acetylated under acidic conditions that also removed the less hindered ketal protecting group. The tetraacetate was reacted with an allyl silane in the presence of BF$_3$•Et$_2$O, producing a β,γ-unsaturated ester via stereoselective allylation on the less hindered face of an oxocarbenium intermediate (Figure 5.34B). Exposure of this triacetate to sodium methoxide in methanol resulted in removal of the acetyl groups, conjugation of the double bond, and oxy-Michael cyclization (Figure 5.34C) that produced a tetrahydropyran with three equatorial substituents. The vicinal diol was oxidatively cleaved with NaIO$_4$ to give an aldehyde, which was subjected to a stereoselective NHK coupling to a 2-bromovinylsilane to give an allylic alcohol. This addition reaction proceeded through a Felkin–Anh transition state wherein the chiral carbon adjacent to the carbonyl controls the developing stereochemistry (Figure 5.34D), producing the anti diastereomer selectively. Note the distinction

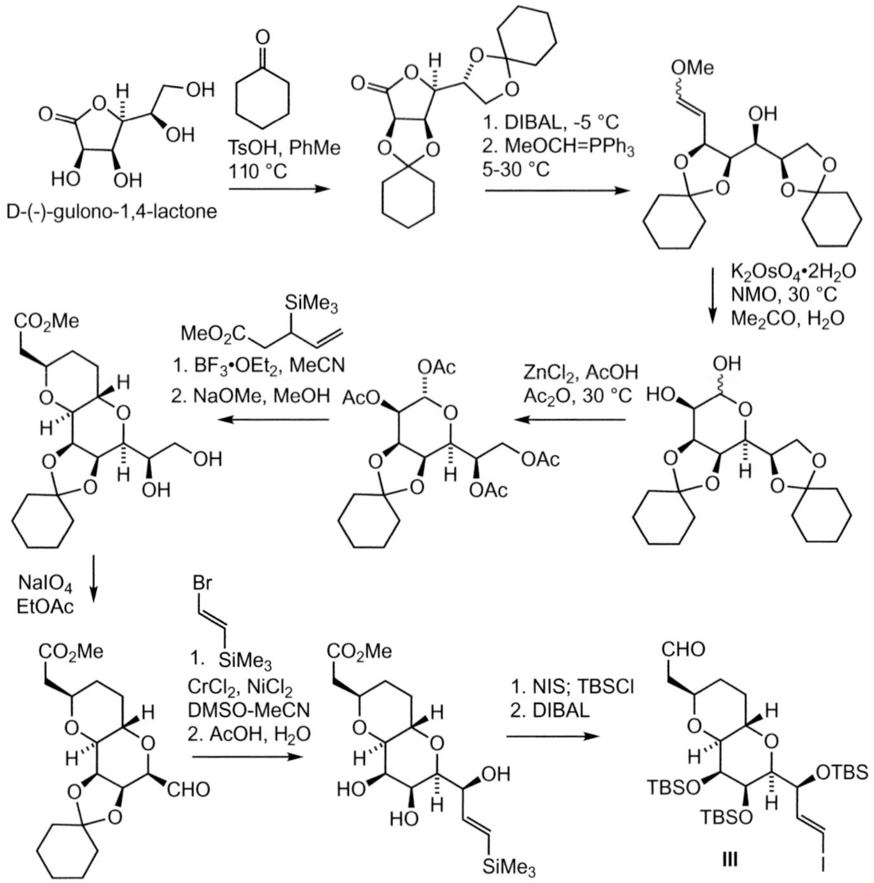

FIGURE 5.33. Synthesis of building block **III**.

between this reaction and the catalytic asymmetric NHK reaction used to synthesize building block **II**, in which case the configuration of the chiral ligand controlled the developing stereochemistry.

With building blocks **I–III** in hand, all that was left to do was to stitch these pieces together. The sequence of reactions that was used to accomplish this is shown in Figure 3.35. First, building block **I** was coupled to building block **II** using the asymmetric catalytic NHK Variant B. The resulting secondary alcohol was deprotonated using potassium hexamethyldisilazide (HMDS), and the alkoxide displaced the mesylate, yielding the C14–C35 backbone of eribulin. This compound was subjected to a Julia-type reaction by deprotonating the sulfone with ^{n}BuLi and reacting the resulting nucleophile with building block **III**, yielding a mixture of β-hydroxy sulfones. The pivalate group was also removed in this step. The resulting diastereomeric diols were oxidized with the Dess–Martin periodinane (DMP) reagent to give

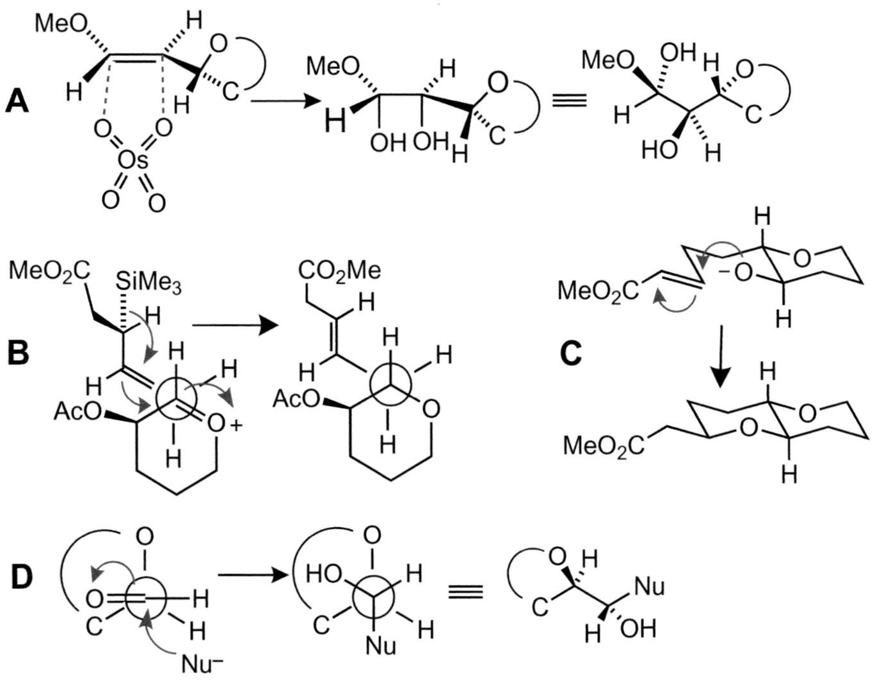

FIGURE 5.34. Rationales for the stereoselectivities observed during the synthesis of building block **III**.

a single β-ketosulfone aldehyde, at which point the sulfone was removed by reductive cleavage with SmI_2. Macrocyclization was accomplished via a ligand-accelerated NHK reaction that linked the vinyl iodide at C13 with the aldehyde at C14 chemoselectively. The resulting mixture of diastereomeric allylic alcohols was oxidized to an enone with the DMP. The final stage of the synthesis began with removal of the five TBS protecting groups with buffered tetrabutylammonium fluoride. An oxo-Michael reaction between the C9 alcohol and the β-carbon of the enone produced a tetrahydrofuran ring. Upon treatment with the mild acid pyridinium para-toluene sulfonate (PPTS), the alcohols at C10 and C11 were perfectly poised to form a ketal, with the carbonyl at C13 producing the desired caged ring system. The terminal diol was then converted to an epoxide by treatment with mesyl chloride and base, and the epoxide was converted to eribulin by ammonolysis.

Given the molecule's size and complexity, the production scale synthesis of eribulin (sold as its mesylate under the brand name Halaven) represents a synthesis milestone. The effort brought together academic and industrial labs to work on a project that, to many, seemed impossible. The synthesis showcased the NHK coupling reaction, which simplified the disconnections that enabled the connection of complex building blocks at the advanced stages of the synthesis. Many of the strategies described in Chapter 1 were used effectively, but the synthesis could not be described

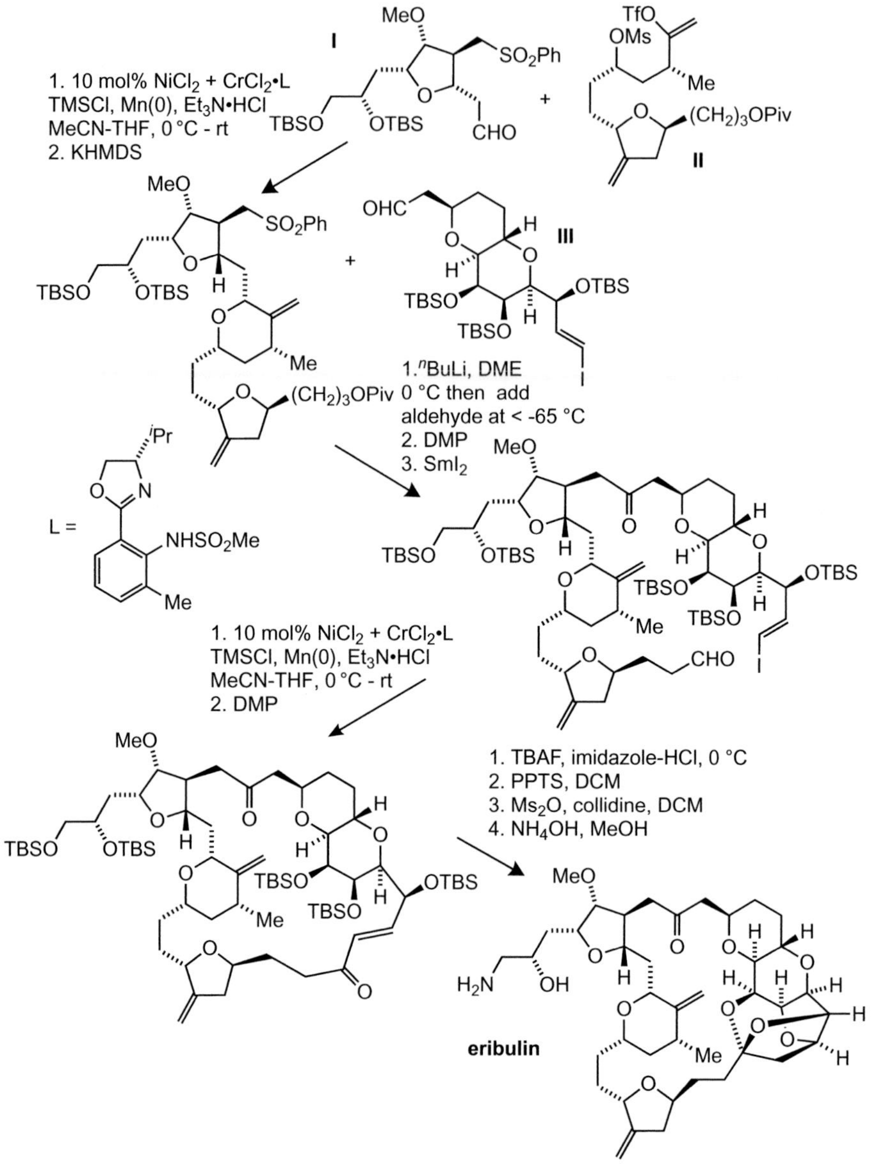

FIGURE 5.35. Final steps in Eisai Pharmaceutical's production scale synthesis of eribulin.

as efficient. Could the synthesis of this complex molecule be made more efficient? This may be considered a challenge for the next generation of synthetic chemists.

SUMMARY

This chapter discussed the synthesis of the polyketide antibiotics erythronolide B, epothilone A, discodermolide, and bahamaolide A and concluded with the production scale synthesis of the anticancer drug eribulin. We started out with Corey's synthesis of erythronolide B, discussing the retrosynthetic analysis of this target and then the actual synthesis and its efficiency. This was followed by the synthesis of epothilone A, first discussing options that could be used to form the 16-membered macrocycle and then detailing Nicolaou's metathesis-based synthesis. Next, the large-scale synthesis of discodermolide was presented, showing that multistep total syntheses can be performed on a process scale. This was followed by an iterative synthesis of the 36-membered macrolide bahamaolide. This synthesis provided an opportunity to introduce the unique chemistry of boronic esters. Finally, the production scale synthesis of the antitumor drug eribulin was presented. The chapter introduced a number of important synthetic methods for building up the carbon skeleton while, at the same time, controlling the stereocenters present in these target molecules. The following short tutorial provides an opportunity to use the concepts that were covered in this chapter to develop a synthetic plan for a typical polyketide. Practice problems that reinforce these concepts will follow.

TUTORIAL: DEVELOPING A SYNTHETIC PLAN FOR A TYPICAL POLYKETIDE STRUCTURE

This short tutorial will show you how to apply some of the tools that have been introduced in this chapter and the previous chapters to a typical polyketide synthesis problem. The target consists of an 18-membered macrocyclic lactone that contains seven stereocenters, three ketones, and a trisubstituted alkene. Our approach will be illustrated retrosynthetically. We are going to use an iterative aldol strategy to generate the stereocenters as we build up the molecule. The overall strategy will be largely **transform-based**.

 Step 1. Identify functional groups in the target molecule noting if they activate proximal carbon atoms. The target molecule has a lactone, three ketones, two alcohols, a methyl ether, and an alkene positioned so that every ring carbon is potentially activable.

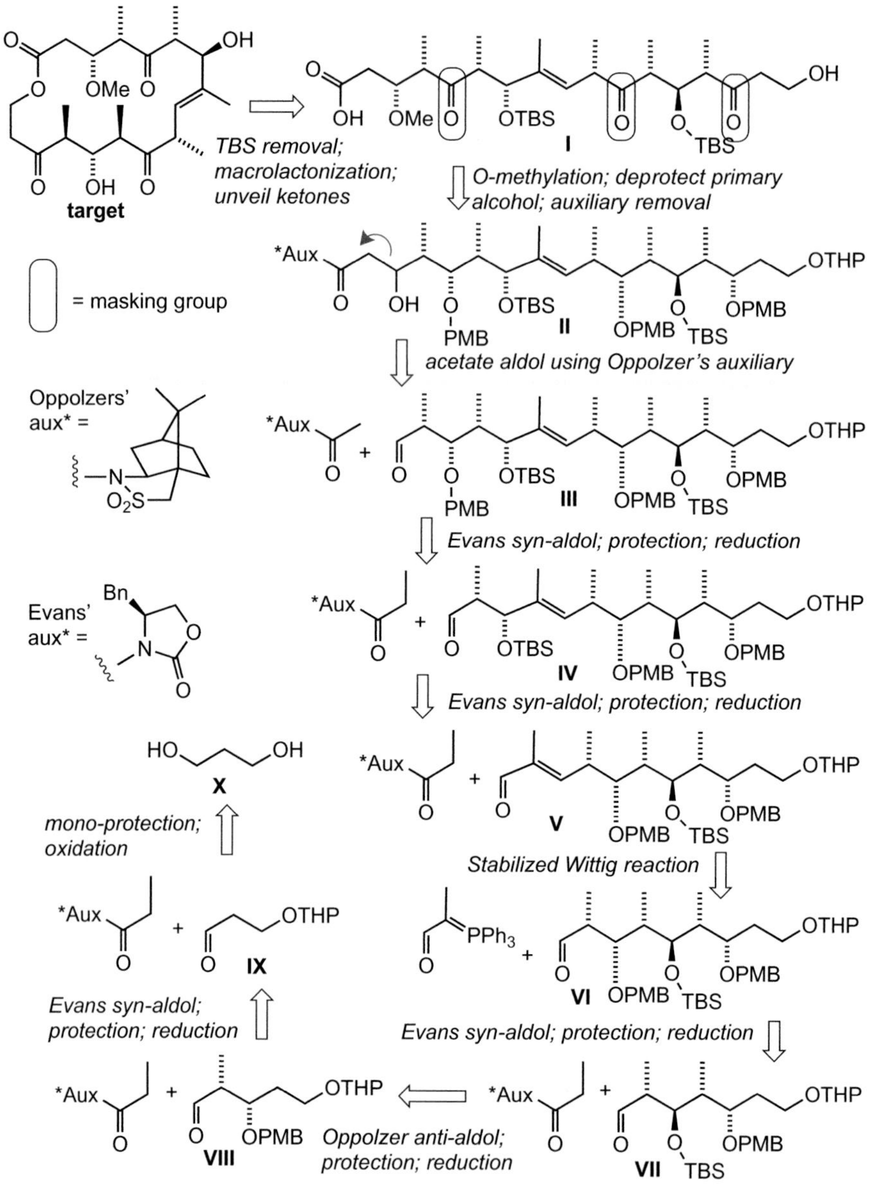

Step 2. Identify patterns that employ powerful transforms or readily available starting materials. If necessary, add functional groups to create powerful retrons. The repeating 1,3-oxygenation pattern suggests that an iterative aldol strategy or its equivalent could be used.

Step 3. Continue your analysis until you reach readily available starting materials. Let's begin by making the standard macrolactone disconnection. This produces a linear molecule that has a carboxylic acid at one end (C1) and a primary alcohol at the other end (C17) of a 17-membered carbon chain. The secondary alcohols at C7 and C13 must be protected to prevent undesired lactonizations. Although there is some flexibility as to exactly which protecting group should be used, the TBS ether is a reasonable choice. The alcohols should be protected so that they do not interfere with these enolate-based reactions and the macrolactonization.

Likewise, the ketones need to be protected to prevent epimerization of the adjacent chiral centers and undesired retro-aldol reactions. One possibility involves masking the three ketones as protected secondary alcohols until after the macrolactonization is completed. At that point, the alcohols C5, C11, and C15 can be revealed and oxidized to ketones. Because these carbons will start out as secondary alcohols formed during aldol homologation, we will leave them in this oxidation state and protect the alcohols as PMB ethers, which will be orthogonal to the TBS protecting groups. In this way, removal of the PMB groups in the presence of the TBS ethers and oxidation of the resultant alcohols can be accomplished once at the end of the synthesis. Oxidizing the alcohols as they are generated would not only add two steps to each iteration but, more importantly, would also result in labile 1,3-dicarbonyl structures that are prone to epimerization. Four reactions are required to go from Structure **II** to the **target** and three reactions to go from **II** to **I**.

Next, we need to decide on the overall strategy for homologation of the growing carbon skeleton. Let's try an aldol addition approach using chiral enolates. Breaking the C2–C3 bond heterolytically places a negative charge on a carbon α to a carbonyl and a positive charge on a methoxy substituted carbon, both of which are stabilizing interactions through resonance and inductive effects. Note that to start from the other end, we would first need to convert the C15 ketone into a carboxylic acid derivative, adding steps to the synthesis. The first asymmetric aldol transform that forms the C1–C2 bond involves an acetic acid-derived enolate, a species that we have not yet seen. Chiral enolates derived from acetimides that incorporate Evans oxazolidinones do not add to aldehydes with high facial selectivity because they lack an important steric interaction present in the propionimide system. However, a reaction that shows good selectivity with the Oppolzer auxiliary has been reported.[7a] This method (based on the work of Teruaki Mukaiyama)[16] involves a silyl ketene acetal and its reaction with an activated aldehyde via an open transition state. Three reactions are used to go from intermediate **III** to **II**.

Now, to build C2–C7, we apply two consecutive propionyl aldol homologations: (1) Evans syn-aldol addition, (2) protection of the alcohol, and (3) conversion of the carboximide into an aldehyde. The (S)-phenylalanine derived oxazolidinone described in the chapter can also be used. A total of six reactions are used to go from intermediate **V** to **III**. One of the virtues of the Evans auxiliary is that the auxiliary-induced stereocontrol generally overrides the existing chirality of the aldehyde.

The (E)-trisubstituted alkene will be introduced stereoselectively via a Wittig reaction that employs a stabilized phosphonium ylide. This reaction is followed by another Evans syn-aldol sequence to introduce C10–C11, but now we are confronted with a new problem: the next aldol homologation (**VIII** to **VII**) must introduce two stereocenters that have the anti relationship at C12–C13. Although there are other methods that can accomplish this, we will use one that is also based on Oppolzer's auxiliary.[7b] The penultimate step in this retrosynthetic analysis involves the application of an Evans syn-aldol reaction with a THP-protected 3-hydroxypropionaldehyde **IX** to install C14–C15. This starting aldehyde can be prepared from 1,3-propane diol **X** by oxidation of the mono-THP ether. Barring unforeseen difficulties, we now have the makings of a viable synthesis plan in place that could be followed empirically.

Note that this retrosynthetic analysis corresponds to just one of many possible branches that make up an inverted synthesis tree. When it comes to designing a synthesis, there is not a unique correct answer. However, some of the branches (synthetic plans) will be more likely to succeed than others. This can be seen when individual students in a group setting work on the same synthesis problem and then each member presents their proposed synthesis to the group for constructive critical feedback. Inevitably, this sort of exercise will result in discussions about the structure and reactivity of molecules. The author believes that this sort of exercise is the best way to learn how to plan a synthesis.

REFERENCES

1. *Perspectives in Organic Chemistry*, Todd, A., Ed., Interscience Publishers: New York 1956, p.155.
2. (a) Corey, E. J., Trybulski, E. J., Melvin Jr., L. S., Nicolaou, K. C., Secrist, J. A., Lett, R., … Brunelle, D. J. (1978). Total synthesis of erythromycins. 3. Stereoselective routes to intermediates corresponding to C (1) to C (9) and C (10) to C (13) fragments of erythronolide B. *Journal of the American Chemical Society, 100*(14), 4618–4620. (b) Corey, E. J., Kim, S., Yoo, S. E., Nicolaou, K. C., Melvin Jr., L. S., Brunelle, D. J., … Sheldrake, P. W. (1978). Total synthesis of erythromycins. 4. Total synthesis of erythronolide B. *Journal of the American Chemical Society, 100*(14), 4620–4622.
3. (a) Yang, Z., He, Y., Vourloumis, D., Vallberg, H., & Nicolaou, K. C. (1997). Total synthesis of epothilone A: The olefin metathesis approach. *Angewandte Chemie International Edition in English, 36*(1–2), 166–168. (b) Nicolaou, K. C., Ninkovic, S., Sarabia, F., Vourloumis, D., He, Y., Vallberg, H., … Yang, Z. (1997). Total syntheses of epothilones A and B via a macrolactonization-based strategy. *Journal of the American Chemical Society, 119*(34), 7974–7991. (c) Nicolaou, K., Winssinger, N., Pastor, J., Ninkovic, S., Sarabia, F., He, Y., … Hamel, E. (1997). Synthesis of epothilones A and B in solid and solution phase. *Nature, 387*(6630), 268–272. https://doi.org/10.1038/387268a0
4. Meng, D., Bertinato, P., Balog, A., Su, D. S., Kamenecka, T., Sorensen, E. J., & Danishefsky, S. J. (1997). Total syntheses of epothilones A and B. *Journal of the American Chemical Society, 119*(42), 10073–10092.
5. Schinzer, D., Limberg, A., Bauer, A., Böhm, O. M., & Cordes, M. (1997). Total synthesis of (-)-epothilone A. *Angewandte Chemie International Edition in English, 36*(5), 523–524.
6. Fürstner, A., Mathes, C., & Lehmann, C. W. (2001). Alkyne metathesis: Development of a novel molybdenum-based catalyst system and its application to the total synthesis of epothilone A and C. *Chemistry–A European Journal, 7*(24), 5299–5317.
7. (a) Oppolzer, W., & Starkemann, C. (1992). Optically pure, crystalline 'acetate'-aldols from N-acetylbornane-10, 2-sultam. *Tetrahedron Letters, 33*(18), 2439–2442. (b) Oppolzer, W., Starkemann, C., Rodriguez, I., & Bernardinelli, G. (1991).

Enantiomerically pure, crystalline 'anti'-aldols from N-acylbornanesultams: Aldolization and structure of intermediate t-butyldimethylsilyl-N, O-ketene acetal. *Tetrahedron Letters*, *32*(1), 61–64.

8. (a) Mickel, S. J., Sedelmeier, G. H., Niederer, D., Daeffler, R., Osmani, A., Schreiner, K., … Xue, S. (2004). Large-scale synthesis of the anti-cancer marine natural product (+)-discodermolide. Part 1: synthetic strategy and preparation of a common precursor. *Organic Process Research and Development*, *8*(1), 92–100. (b) Mickel, S. J., Sedelmeier, G. H., Niederer, D., Schuerch, F., Grimler, D., Koch, G., … Waykole, L. (2004). Large-scale synthesis of the anti-cancer marine natural product (+)-discodermolide. Part 2: Synthesis of fragments C1-6 and C9-14. *Organic Process Research and Development*, *8*(1), 101–106. (c) Mickel, S. J., Sedelmeier, G. H., Niederer, D., Schuerch, F., Koch, G., Kuesters, E., … Waykole, L. (2004). Large-scale synthesis of the anti-cancer marine natural product (+)-discodermolide. Part 3: synthesis of fragment C15-21. *Organic Process Research and Development*, *8*(1), 107–112. (d) Mickel, S. J., Sedelmeier, G. H., Niederer, D., Schuerch, F., Seger, M., Schreiner, K., … Paterson, I. (2004). Large-scale synthesis of the anti-cancer marine natural product (+)-discodermolide. Part 4: Preparation of fragment C7-24. *Organic Process Research and Development*, *8*(1), 113–121. (e) Mickel, S. J., Niederer, D., Daeffler, R., Osmani, A., Kuesters, E., Schmid, E., … Paterson, I. (2004). Large-scale synthesis of the anti-cancer marine natural product (+)-discodermolide. Part 5: Linkage of fragments C1-6 and C7-24 and finale. *Organic Process Research and Development*, *8*(1), 122–130.

9. Evans, D. A., Takacs, J. M., McGee, L. R., Ennis, M. D., Mathre, D. J., & Bartroli, J. (1981). Chiral enolate design. *Pure and Applied Chemistry*, *53*(6), 1109–1127.

10. Chemler, S. R., Trauner, D., & Danishefsky, S. J. (2001). The B-Alkyl Suzuki–Miyaura cross-coupling reaction: Development, mechanistic study, and applications in natural product synthesis. *Angewandte Chemie International Edition*, *40*(24), 4544–4568.

11. Hiyama, T., Okude, Y., Kimura, K., & Nozaki, H. (1982). Highly selective carbon-carbon bond forming reactions mediated by chromium (II) reagents. *Bulletin of the Chemical Society of Japan*, *55*(2), 561–568.

12. Aiken, S. G., Bateman, J. M., Liao, H. H., Fawcett, A., Bootwicha, T., Vincetti, P., … Aggarwal, V. K. (2022). Iterative synthesis of 1, 3-polyboronic esters with high stereocontrol and application to the synthesis of bahamaolide A. *Nature Chemistry 15*(2), 248–256.

13. Bauer, A. (2016). Story of eribulin mesylate: Development of the longest drug synthesis. In: Časar, Z., Ed., *Synthesis of heterocycles in contemporary medicinal chemistry. Topics in heterocyclic chemistry, 44*, 209–270.

14. Gil, A., Albericio, F., & Alvarez, M. (2017). Role of the Nozaki–Hiyama–Takai–Kishi reaction in the synthesis of natural products. *Chemical Reviews*, *117*(12), 8420–8446.

15. Tokunaga, M., Larrow, J. F., Kakiuchi, F., & Jacobsen, E. N. (1997). Asymmetric catalysis with water: Efficient kinetic resolution of terminal epoxides by means of catalytic hydrolysis. *Science*, *277*(5328), 936–938.

16. Kan, S. J., Ng, K. K. H., & Paterson, I. (2013). The impact of the Mukaiyama aldol reaction in total synthesis. *Angewandte Chemie International Edition*, *52*(35), 9097–9108.

PRACTICE PROBLEMS

1. How might one modify the synthetic sequences in Figures 5.4 and 5.6 to make the synthesis of erythronolide B enantioselective, thus avoiding the need for a resolution and the wasteful production of an unwanted diastereomer?

2. Design an enantioselective synthesis of the following molecule from building blocks of five or fewer carbons.

3. Perform a retrosynthetic analysis on the seco-acid of 6-deoxyerythronolide B using Evans's syn-selective asymmetric aldol addition methodology and Oppolzer's asymmetric alkylation methodology to set the stereocenters.

4. Design a stereocontrolled synthesis of the following molecule.

5. Referring to the retrosynthetic analysis that was presented in this chapter's tutorial and **Step 4** in the holistic approach, write out a forward synthetic plan (including reagents) as a series of organic reactions that would lead to the target molecule.

Index

Note: Page numbers in *italics* indicate figures